The Calorie Guide to Branded Foods

The Calorie Guide to Branded Foods

by ALEXANDRA SHERMAN

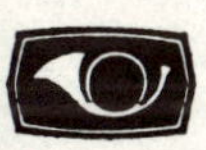

Arlington Books
King Street, St. James's
London

THE CALORIE GUIDE TO
BRANDED FOODS

*first published 1979 by
Arlington Books (Publishers) Ltd
15–17 King Street
London SW1*

*revised edition July 1984
second impression November 1984
third impression December 1985*

© *1984 Alexandra Sherman*

*Typeset by Preface Ltd, Salisbury
Printed and bound by
The Bath Press, Bath*

ISBN 85140 307 7

Acknowledgements

Once again the author has been most impressed by the helpfulness of nearly all the companies approached. Most replied immediately to requests for information and were happy to supply the necessary figures, if available. It is particularly regretted not to be able to include the Sharwood range of Indian products but sadly the manufacturer did not seem able to supply the information at the time of going to press. Bejam—the freezer-food specialists—were very helpful but are presently in the process of analysing their 'own brand' lines and were therefore only able to supply calorie-figures for a limited range of their products at this time. It is hoped that many more of their products will be included in the next edition. Marks and Spencer were, as always, extremely cooperative but pointed out that they change their range of products with such frequency that it would never be possible to supply completely up-to-date lists of foods available on their shelves. The reason for the omission of Sainsbury from this edition is that they publish their own little booklet entitled *Balancing Your Diet* which lists the protein, fat, calorie and carbohydrate content of all their products.

Contents

Foreword to Second Edition

This edition has been completely up-dated which means that no figures were taken from the first edition. All have been obtained direct from the manufacturers.

There has been a staggering increase in the number of products on the food market since publication of the last edition of this book five years ago. This is particularly true of ready-prepared meals and frozen foods. One can now buy an incredible range of British, French, Italian, Chinese, Indian and even Mexican dishes—either ready to eat or in the form of sauce mixes. As many of these as possible have been included which should ensure that any diet embarked on using this book will certainly not lack variety!

To make it feasible to include so many new products without greatly increasing the length of the book, some sections have had to be reduced. This has been achieved by amalgamating items where all brands have approximately the same calorie-content. This applies mainly in the biscuits, cereals and drinks sections. In the vegetable section many previously included which have less than 25 calories per 100 g, are not in this new edition.

Shops specializing in 'Health Foods' have mushroomed all over the country in the past few years and we are happy to be able to include quite a wide range of these products in this new edition. This also means the inclusion of quite a number of foodstuffs (dairy-substitutes, for example) suitable for vegetarians.

You will probably have heard of the advantages of a high-fibre diet for quick, healthy weight loss. Although this book does not list the fibre content of foods it will certainly be useful to those on a high-fibre diet. The author personally feels that eating extra fibre *does* assist weight-loss and certainly is healthy so do try to pick products which are known to be high in fibre. Having said that, however, it must be said that this book is still aimed at those of you who want to lose weight but do not like being told what to eat and what not to eat. This book is for those who prefer to 'do their own thing'.

Foreword

This little book is aimed primarily at those people—
and there are many of us—who always have had
and probably always will have what is euphemisti-
cally called a 'weight problem'. There are—alas—
very few people who can eat whatever they want, in
any quantity, without putting on weight. The idea
behind this book is that, when used in conjunction
with *The Pocket Calorie Guide to Safe Slimming* by
Jane Colin, you can eat what you like but easily
regulate the quantity to ensure that no weight is
gained. It will also, of course, be invaluable to those
who have a great deal of weight to lose—nothing is
more boring than weeks on end eating only cottage
cheese and grapefruit! With this book to help you,
there is no reason why you shouldn't have, for
example, a piece of cake for tea, as long as it is carefully weighed and the calories included with your
allowance for the day. In this book you will be able
to find the actual brand name of the piece of cake
you wish to eat, so no mistakes need be made; after
all, 'one medium slice of chocolate cake' could
mean different things to different people. That is
why—where possible—weights have been given

per ounce and per hundred grammes, so that every-
thing can be properly weighed and there is no
excuse for cheating. One exception is biscuits, since
most of the manufacturers in this category supplied
only the figures per biscuit, and it was therefore
necessary to list them in this way.

It must be stressed that before embarking on
any diet you should confirm with your doctor that
you are in good health. For somebody who is very
overweight it can be a considerable shock to the
system to reduce the calorie intake drastically, so
please tell your doctor what you are planning to do.
In most cases doctors will approve wholeheartedly.
At this point I should add that, although the figures
quoted are quite accurate enough for a weight loss
diet, they should not be used by anybody who must
limit or avoid any particular food-stuff for medical
reasons.

It is advisable to go out and buy a good,
accurate pair of scales. I find the type used for mail
to be extremely useful. It can be all too easy to
cheat using ordinary kitchen scales!

So, you have this book, and probably another
book which lists the calorie content of foods in their
natural state, and you are all set to get your weight
down to its correct level (there is a table at the end
of the Foreword giving average weights for men and
women). To do this, you must find out by trial and
error to what level you, personally, must reduce

your intake of calories in order to achieve your required weight loss per week (always think in terms of per week, and not per day, as it can be very depressing to weigh yourself daily since you cannot expect to lose every day). This level should never go below 750 calories per day if you are leading a normal life. It is fine to starve yourself for a couple of days if you are able to relax and do nothing—but this is not the way to achieve a permanent weight loss. In any case this particular book is certainly not for those who wish to starve themselves, but rather for those who want to be able to eat what they enjoy, and enjoy what they eat!

Most *average* people will achieve a satisfactory weight loss (I must stress *average*, as each body is different) on 1000 calories per day for women, and 1200–1500 per day for men. But even on 500 more than that per day respectively, you will still lose weight, albeit slowly. Once your desired weight is reached, in order to avoid gaining weight a satisfactory daily allowance is 2250 calories for most women, and slightly more for most men. But, and this cannot be repeated too often, each person is different, and to begin with it has to be a case of trial and error. If you find you are gaining weight on 2250 calories per day then you must reduce the daily allowance and try again.

This little calorie guide can be used by anybody—either to lose weight or, once this has been achieved, to maintain the ideal figure. The causes and effects of obesity are gone into in greater detail in Jane Colin's *New Pocket Calorie Guide to Safe Slimming*, but there is only one possible cure— *eat less*. With this book this should be fairly easy without too much suffering. Good luck!

You may wonder why no so-called "slimming foods" have been included in this book. This was a calculated decision. The nutritional content (including calories) of all such foods is carefully listed on the packaging and, as we want to keep this *pocket* book as concise as possible, we feel it to be unnecessary to include them.

The figures given have been supplied by the manufacturers very recently but, unfortunately, it may be that by the time the book is published some of the products will have been discontinued and other new ones will have appeared. This is unavoidable, and the tables will be updated as often as possible for each new edition. It is also impossible to list every food-stuff available in Britain, but if you find a particular brand-name food missing you will probably be able to find an equivalent under a different name. Although this is by no means ideal, it is better to use the figures from another brand-name than not to count the calories at all!

WHAT YOU SHOULD WEIGH

The following weight table is of necessity only average. Each person has an ideal weight at which they look and feel their best. A person with large bones can weigh as much as half a stone more than somebody with small bones and still look very good. The best way to find out whether you are large, medium or small boned is to measure your wrist (and no cheating!).

For women: wrists measuring $5\frac{1}{2}''$ mean small bones; $6-6\frac{1}{2}''$ mean medium bones; over $6\frac{1}{2}''$ mean large bones.

For men: wrists measuring $6\frac{1}{2}''-7''$ mean small bones; $7-7\frac{1}{2}''$ mean medium bones; over $8''$ mean large bones.

So use the following tables only as a guideline. Those of you with small or large bones should deduct or add between five and seven pounds (two to three kilos) from these weights.

AVERAGE WEIGHTS TABLE

(These weights include no clothes. For light clothing but no shoes you should add three pounds (1.4 kilos)).

MEN						WOMEN				
Height			*Weight*			*Height*			*Weight*	
Ft.	*Ins.*	*St.*	*Lbs.*	*Kilos*		*Ft.*	*Ins.*	*St.*	*Lbs.*	*Kilos*
5	0	8	10	55.5		4	8	7	8	48.2
5	1	8	12	56.4		4	9	7	10	49.1
5	2	9	0	57.3		4	10	7	12	50.0
5	3	9	3	58.6		4	11	8	0	50.9
5	4	9	6	60.0		5	0	8	2	51.8
5	5	9	10	61.8		5	1	8	4	52.7
5	6	10	0	63.6		5	2	8	6	53.6
5	7	10	4	65.5		5	3	8	11	55.9
5	8	10	8	67.3		5	4	8	13	56.8
5	9	10	12	69.1		5	5	9	2	58.2
5	10	11	3	71.4		5	6	9	6	60.0
5	11	11	8	73.6		5	7	9	10	61.8
6	0	12	0	76.4		5	8	10	0	63.6
6	1	12	6	79.1		5	9	10	4	65.5
6	2	12	12	81.8		5	10	10	8	67.3
6	3	13	4	84.5		5	11	10	11	68.6
6	4	13	10	87.3		6	0	11	1	70.5

Biscuits—Sweet, Plain

Sweet biscuits are high in calories and of not much nutritional value. Nevertheless to relax with a cup of coffee and a biscuit or two is very comforting after several days of stringent dieting. This you can do without exceeding your daily calorie allowance with the help of the following tables. Chocolate biscuits should be avoided except very occasionally because, as can be seen, some have as many calories as a bar of chocolate.

Food	Quantities	Calories
Miscellaneous		
Custard Cream	1 biscuit	65
Digestive	,,	65
Fruit Shortcake	,,	40
Ginger Nut	,,	40
Lincoln	,,	40
Marie	,,	30
Morning Coffee ..	,,	25
Nice	,,	45
Rich Tea, round ..	,,	40
Rich Tea, finger ..	,,	25

Food	Quantities	Calories
ALLINSON		
Bran Oatcakes	1 biscuit	50
Scottish Shortbread	,,	85
'Hand Baked'–Bran	,,	65
,, –Coconut	,,	70
,, –Demerara	,,	65
,, –Fruit & Nut	,,	64
,, –Ginger	,,	49
,, –Hazelnut	,,	63
,, –Honey	,,	57
,, –Muesli	,,	60
,, –Oatmeal	,,	61
,, –Peanut	,,	61
,, –Walnut	,,	65
CRAWFORD		
Balmoral	1 biscuit	8
'Pennywise' Finger Nice	,,	28
,, Finger Tea	,,	21
,, Garibaldi	,,	33
,, Iced Shorties	,,	40
,, Jam Rings	,,	62
,, Lemon Creams	,,	58
,, Malties	,,	37
,, Orange Creams	,,	58
,, Raspberry Creams	,,	47
,, Shortcake	,,	59
,, Shorties	,,	37
Petticoat Tail	,,	57
Shortbread Highland Finger	,,	63
Tartan Shortbread	,,	97
Thin Arrowroot	,,	30

Food	Quantities	Calories
HUNTLEY AND PALMER		
Barbary	1 biscuit	51
Braemar	,,	29
Burford	,,	60
Fruit Digestive	,,	50
Gingerella	,,	28
Sponge Finger	,,	21
Wafer Delight	,,	97
INTERNATIONAL		
Coconut Cookie	1 oz	140
Coconut Crumble Cream	,,	149
Coffee Cream	,,	130
Fig Roll	,,	100
Garibaldi	,,	103
Lemon Puff Cream	,,	142
Malted Milk	,,	138
Orange Cream	,,	130
Rich Shorties	,,	141
Shortcake	,,	145
MACFARLANE LANG		
Abernethy	1 biscuit	60
Granola	,,	57
MCVITIE 'COUNTRY COOKIES'		
Almond & Honey	1 biscuit	86
Cherry & Coconut	,,	79
Hazelnut & Raisin	,,	82
MCVITIE		
Abbey Crunch	1 biscuit	47
Crumblebake Creams	,,	92
Digestive Creams	,,	74

Food	Quantities	Calories
Fruit 'n' spice	1 biscuit	35
Fruit Shortcake	,,	50
Gypsy Creams	,,	83
Golden Crumble ..	,,	40
Royal Scot	,,	53
Wheatmeal	,,	73

MARKS AND SPENCER

Food	Quantities	Calories
Almond	1 biscuit	49
All Butter	,,	46
Brandy Snap	,,	24
Butter Crunch	,,	33
Butter Crunch Cream ..	,,	67
Crunch Sandwich ..	,,	65
Curls	,,	38
Dutch Finger Creams ..	,,	48
Fruit Shortcake	1 oz	135
Jam Sandwich	1 biscuit	71
Meringue Nests	,,	61
Muesli	,,	79
Oatflake and Apple ..	,,	76
Shortbread Fingers ..	,,	109
Shorties	,,	54
Sultana	,,	75

MITCHELLHILL

Food	Quantities	Calories
Healthy Life	1 biscuit	61
Honey Wheaten ..	,,	61
Oatcakes & Bran ..	,,	50

PEAK FREAN

Food	Quantities	Calories
Coffee Cream	1 biscuit	57
Country Crunch ..	,,	30
Crunch Cream	,,	57

Food	Quantities	Calories
Currant Crisp	1 biscuit	30
Devon Cream	,,	53
Garibaldi	,,	30
Iced Gem	,,	3
Jaffa Crunch	,,	30
Jersey Cream	,,	57
Malty	,,	39
Neapolitan Wafer ..	,,	37
Orange Cream	,,	57
Rich Osborne	,,	35
Shortcake	,,	51
Treacle Crunch	,,	29

PREWETT

Food	Quantities	Calories
Carob Chip	1 biscuit	65
Fig	,,	60
Sesame & Sunflower ..	,,	66
Stem Ginger	,,	59
Wholemeal	,,	64

SPAR

Food	Quantities	Calories
Big 5 Caramel Wafer ..	1 oz	136
Coconut Crumble Cream ..	,,	149
Fig Roll	,,	109
Garibaldi	,,	103
Ginger Thin	,,	133
Jam Rings	,,	132
Lemon Crumble Cream ..	,,	145
Lemon Puff	,,	144
Majestic Wafer	,,	131
Shortbread Finger ..	,,	147
Shortcake	,,	145
Shorties	,,	139
Strawberry Crumble Cream	,,	147

Food	Quantities	Calories
Teacake	1 oz	132
Vanilla Wafer	„	148
TESCO		
All Butter Thin	1 oz	133
Butter Ring	„	151
Caramel Cookies	„	146
Caramel Wafer	„	135
Coconut Crumble	„	149
Coconut Macaroon	„	135
Coconut Rings	„	149
Coffee	„	130
Cookie Crunch	„	127
Digestive, cream filled	„	145
Garibaldi	„	115
Jam–Cream Sandwich	„	135
Jam–Sandwich	„	133
Jam Tarts, mini	„	132
Lemon Crispy & Crumble	„	143
Malted Milk	„	145
Oatmeal Cookies, mini	„	133
Orange	„	138
Rich Shortie	„	142
Shortbread Finger	„	146
Shortcakes, plain	„	142
Shortcakes, petticoat	„	145
WAITROSE		
Biscuits, assorted	1 oz	158
Butter Crunch	„	129
Coconut Cookies	„	141
Coconut Cream	„	145
Cream Biscuits, assorted	„	142
Danish Shortcake	„	150

Food	Quantities	Calories
Fruit Shortcake	1 oz	143
Garibaldi	,,	108
Iced Ring	,,	127
Gingerbread Men ..	,,	126
Malted Milk Bears ..	,,	132
Scotch Butter Shortbread ..	,,	148
Shortbread Fingers ..	,,	148
Shortcake	,,	143
Sultana Cookies ..	,,	136

Biscuits—Chocolate

Food	Quantities	Calories
Miscellaneous		
Bourbon	1 biscuit	65
Chocolate Chip	,,	55
Chocolate Digestive ..	,,	70
Chocolate Wheatmeal ..	,,	80
Jaffa	,,	50
CADBURY		
Animals	1 biscuit	30
Bournville		
Oval	,,	55
Ring	,,	60
Sandwich	,,	80
Shamrock	,,	50
Wafer	,,	65
Bournville Digestive ..	,,	45
Coasters & Cookies ..	,,	45
Fingers	,,	25
Milk Assorted		
Oval	,,	55
Ring	,,	60
Sandwich	,,	75
Shamrock	,,	45
Wafer	,,	65
Milk Digestive	,,	50

Food	Quantities	Calories
Orange Creams	1 biscuit	80
Shorties	,,	50
HUNTLEY AND PALMER		
Choc Chip 'n' Nut	1 biscuit	44
Snowball	,,	131
INTERNATIONAL		
Choc 'N' Nut Cookies	1 oz	146
Chocolate Coated Short Cake	,,	30
JACOB		
Club–average all flavours	1 biscuit	110
Coated Mallow, milk & plain	,,	56
MACDONALDS		
54321	1 biscuit	100
Taxi	,,	80
Yo Yo, mint	,,	100
Yo Yo, toffee	,,	93
MCVITIE		
Bandit	1 biscuit	91
Big Bar Bandit	,,	215
Chocolate Biscuit Finger	,,	25
Chocolate Digestive	,,	98
Chocolate Homewheat	,,	84
Chocolate Sports	,,	107
Munchmallow	,,	81
Penguin	,,	125
United Extra Time	,,	223
MARKS AND SPENCER		
Biscuit Thins, plain	1 biscuit	30

Food	Quantities	Calories
Break In	1 biscuit	119
Chocolate Crisp, plain	,,	42
Finger Wafers–milk & plain	,,	44
Milk Caramel Wafers	,,	96
Milk Crunch	,,	34
Mint Sundae	,,	87
Plain Ginger	,,	64
Sponge Mallow	,,	89
Tea Biscuit, milk	,,	72
PEAK FREAN		
Coconut Mallow	1 biscuit	46
Jamboree Mallow	,,	77
SPAR		
Choc 'n' Nut Cookies	1 oz	142
Fully Coated Choc. Finger	,,	148
Mallow-Filled Wafer	,,	72
Milk Choc. Sandwich	,,	148
Snowball	,,	120
TESCO		
Coconut rings, plain	1 oz	134
Dundee	,,	138
Orange	,,	146
Sandwich	,,	148
Shortcake	,,	145
Tea Cakes	,,	121
Wafer	,,	142
WAITROSE		
Plain Chocolate Orange Cream Sandwich	1 oz	147
Wafer Sandwich Biscuits w/Chocolate Filling	,,	143

Biscuits—Savoury

Savoury biscuits may be usefully substituted for bread on a diet but care should be taken to count the calories carefully and not eat too many.

Food	Quantities	Calories
CARR'S		
Water Table, large	1 biscuit	32
Water Table, small	,,	14
CRAWFORDS		
Butter Puff	1 biscuit	50
Cheddar	,,	22
Cheese Savor	,,	3
Cream Cracker	,,	33
TUC	,,	23
TUC Savoury Cream	,,	71
FORTIS		
Bath Oliver	1 biscuit	49
INTERNATIONAL		
Biscuits for Cheese	1 oz	120
Cheese Thins	,,	152
Cream Cracker	,,	125
Light Crispbread	,,	111
Savoury Sticks	,,	120

Food	Quantities	Calories
JACOBS		
Cheese & Onion sandwich ..	1 biscuit	47
Cornish Wafer	,,	44
Cream Cracker	,,	33
Water Biscuits/High Bake ..	,,	31
MARKS AND SPENCER		
Bran Sunnywheat ..	1 biscuit	38
Butter Puff	,,	50
Cheese Sandwich ..	,,	52
Cheese Snap	,,	3
Cream Cracker	,,	37
Light Crispbread ..	,,	17
Wholemeal Bran ..	,,	67
MCVITIE		
Kracka Wheat	1 biscuit	38
Macvita	,,	33
Ry King Crispbread, Fibre		
Plus	,,	28
,, Brown	,,	33
,, Light	,,	24
,, Wheat	,,	34
NABISCO		
Dutch Crispbake ..	1 biscuit	38
Ritz, Cheese & Plain ..	,,	16
SPAR		
Cream Crackers ..	1 oz	123
Wheat Crackers ..	,,	128
TESCO		
Cheese Sandwich ..	1 oz	145

Food		Quantities	Calories
Cheese Savouries	..	1 oz	148
Cheese Thins	.. ..	,,	152
Cornish Wafer	.. ..	,,	156
Cream Cracker	.. ..	,,	129
High Baked Water	..	,,	112
Poppy Sesame Crackers	..	,,	148
Snack Cracker	.. ..	,,	151
Wheat Cracker	.. ..	,,	126
WAITROSE			
Cream Crackers	..	1 oz	130
Savoury Crackers	..	,,	169

Bread, Buns, etc

As the calorific content of the various brands of bread varies only slightly these products have been listed under food rather than brand name. *But*—weigh your slices carefully because the homemade style loaves are much denser and therefore inclined to weigh more. A slice of bread, where indicated on a diet sheet, should weigh approximately 30 g. With homemade 100% wholemeal it is remarkably easy to cut a slice weighing 60 g!

Food	Quantities	Calories	Quantities	Calories
Bath Buns	1 oz	88	100 g	310
Brown Bread	,,	72	,,	254
Brown Bread with Bran	,,	71	,,	250
Crumpets	,,	54	,,	190
Currant Buns (no butter)	,,	90	,,	317
Granary Bread	,,	64	,,	225
'High Protein' Bread	,,	71	,,	250
Malt Loaf	,,	85	,,	300
Scones	,,	90	,,	317
Scotch Pancakes	,,	87	,,	307
White Bread	,,	73	,,	257
100% Wholemeal Bread	,,	78	,,	274

Cakes, Pies, Cake Mixes, Pastries

All products in this section should be avoided by anybody on a serious slimming diet. After all, one slice of cake uses up nearly half the daily allowance of calories. They have been included, however, as it is useful for anybody on a 'maintenance' diet to know the calorific content of even the most fattening foods.

Food	Quantities	Calories	Quantities	Calories
BIRD'S EYE *(frozen)*				
Blackforest Gateau	1/6 of cake	250		
Chocolate Gateau	,,	200		
Cheesecake–Fruit	,,	260		
4 Choux Buns	1 packet	500		
Dairy Cream & Choc. Sponge	1/6 of cake	110		
Dairy Cream Doughnuts	One	170		
Dairy Cream Eclairs	One	130		
Dairy Cream Sponge	1/6 of cake	130		
Dairy Cream Gateau	,,	175		
Strawberry Gateau	,,	280		
Puff Pastry	1 oz	120	100 g	422
Puff Pastry Sheets	1 sheet	360		
Shortcrust Pastry	1 oz	125	100 g	440
Vol au Vent Cases	One	70		

Cakes, Pies, Cake Mixes, Pastries

Food	Quantities	Calories	Quantities	Calories
CADBURY				
Angel Layer Cake ..	1 oz	120	100 g	424
Battenburg	,,	103	,,	363
Battenburg Treats ..	each	172	—	—
Black Forest Gateau ..	1 oz	112	100 g	423
Buttercream Sponge ..	,,	119	,,	418
Buttercream Walnut Cake	,,	122	,,	429
Cherry Fruit Cake ..	,,	87	,,	308
Chocolate Cake ..	,,	112	,,	396
Chocolate Dainties ..	each	125	—	—
Chocolate Fudge Cake ..	1 oz	103	100 g	363
Chocolate Log ..	,,	115	,,	406
Chocolate Sponge Cake ..	,,	98	,,	344
Chocolate Whirls ..	each	129	—	—
Continental Gateau ..	1 oz	120	100 g	423
Corners	each	428	—	—
Flake Cakes	,,	127	—	—
French Fancies, all flavours	,,	105	—	—
French Jam Sponge ..	1 oz	94	100 g	332
Golden Sponge Cake ..	,,	98	,,	347
Jaffa Fingers	each	128	—	—
Jamaica Ginger Cake ..	1 oz	93	100 g	328
Madeira Cake	,,	109	,,	385
Manor House Cake ..	,,	116	,,	410
Mini Rolls	each	113	—	—
Regal Roll	1 oz	87	100 g	307
Swiss Gateau ..	,,	112	,,	396
Swiss Roll	,,	117	,,	413
Victoria Sponge ..	,,	64	,,	224
GRANNYSMITHS				
Bread Roll	1 oz	104	100 g	368

Food	Quantities	Calories	Quantities	Calories
Cheesecake	1 packet	748	—	—
Chocolate Sponge ..	,,	684	—	—
Crumble	1 oz	110	100 g	388
Crunch Base	,,	135	,,	476
Doughnut	,,	103	,,	364
Lemon Madeira Cake ..	1 packet	916	—	—
Luxury Sponge ..	,,	999	—	—
Pizza Base	1 oz	102	100 g	358
Scone	,,	112	,,	396
Shortbread	,,	102	,,	358
Short Pastry	,,	140	,,	493
Short Pastry w/Bran ..	,,	137	,,	484
Spicy Cake	1 pkt	958	—	—
Suet Dumpling ..	1 oz	143	100 g	503
Wheatmeal Bread ..	,,	95	,,	299
White Bread	,,	101	,,	357
Yorkshire Pudding ..	,,	96	,,	338

US ROLL
| Puff Pastry & Vol-au-Vents | 1 oz | 111 | 100 g | 393 |

LYONS
(large cakes)
Battenburg	1 oz	104	100 g	366
Brandy (canned) ..	,,	91	,,	319
Butter Madeira ..	,,	108	,,	380
Chocolate Sponge Slice ..	,,	103	,,	362
'Dessert Harvest Pies'				
Apple	,,	91	,,	322
Apple & Blackcurrant ..	,,	90	,,	316
Dundee (canned) ..	,,	89	,,	315
Flan Case	,,	99	,,	348

Cakes, Pies, Cake Mixes, Pastries

Food	Quantities	Calories	Quantities	Calories
Jamaica Ginger ..	1 oz	93	100 g	328
Queen Victoria Sponge				
(frozen) ..	,,	93	,,	328
'Sponge Rolls'				
Black Currant ..	,,	101	,,	357
Chocolate	,,	114	,,	400
Chocolate	,,	106	,,	373
Jam	,,	85	,,	298
Jam & Vanilla ..	,,	95	,,	333
'Sponge Sandwiches'				
Chocolate	,,	106	,,	373
Coffee	,,	116	,,	408
Jam & Vanilla ..	,,	102	,,	361
Raspberry	,,	93	,,	328
Triple Decker	,,	92	,,	325
Yule Log	,,	115	,,	405
(small cakes)				
Apricot Madeleines ..	Each	114	—	—
Chocolate Caprice ..	,,	140	—	—
'Cup Cakes'				
Chocolate	,,	129	—	—
Orange & Lemon ..	,,	129	—	—
'Fruit Pies'				
Apple	,,	176	—	—
Apple & Blackcurrant ..	,,	176	—	—
'Harvest Pies'	,,			
Apple	,,	355	—	—
Apple & Blackcurrant ..	,,	354	—	—
Apricot	,,	360	—	—
'Iced Tarts'				
Almond	,,	127	—	—
Chocolate	,,	119	—	—

Food	Quantities	Calories	Quantities	Calories
Jam Tarts–all flavours ..	Each	99	—	—
'Junior Chocolate Rolls'				
Caramel	,,	107	—	—
Raspberry	,,	97	—	—
Mince Pies	,,	194	—	—
'Puff Pastries'				
Apple	,,	196	—	—
Apple & Blackcurrant ..	,,	186	—	—
Mince	,,	187	—	—
Trifle Sponges ..	,,	79	—	—
LYONS				
Batter Mix	1 oz	103	100 g	362
Doughnut Mix ..	,,	110	,,	389
Pastry Mix	,,	133	,,	469
Suet Pudding Mix ..	,,	140	,,	493
'Chocolate Baking Aids'				
Melt in the Bag				
Covering ..	,,	163	,,	575
Polka Dots	,,	145	,,	510
MCVITIE				
Cherry Fruit Piece ..	1 oz	93	100 g	328
Cherry Fruit Slab ..	,,	149	,,	524
Cherry Genoa	,,	98	,,	347
Cherry No. 2	,,	95	,,	335
Christmas–Iced Top ..	,,	71	,,	250
Christmas–Marzipan ..	,,	78	,,	276
Chocolate	1/8 cake	140	—	—
Chumbles	each	116	—	—
Dark Orange	1/8 cake	135	—	—
Golden Syrup	,,	142	—	—
Jamaica Ginger ..	,,	134	—	—

Cakes, Pies, Cake Mixes, Pastries

Food	Quantities	Calories	Quantities	Calories
Kensington	1 oz	100	100 g	354
Lemon Spice	1/8 cake	144	—	—
Tunis	1 oz	128	100 g	452
MARKS AND SPENCER				
(large cakes)				
All Butter Madeira or Walnut ..	1 oz	115	100 g	405
All Butter Cherry Genoa ..	,,	93	,,	327
Apple Sponge	,,	68	,,	240
Angel S/W Cut ..	,,	163	,,	574
Battenburg	,,	102	,,	360
Cherry Cut	,,	112	,,	394
Country	,,	115	,,	405
Country Style Cut ..	,,	102	,,	360
Double Layer Sponge ..	,,	77	,,	272
Gingerbread	,,	87	,,	308
Ginger Sandwich ..	,,	114	,,	400
Iced All Butter Madeira S/W ..	,,	110	,,	389
Parkin Cut	,,	93	,,	329
Spiced Raisin	,,	99	,,	348
Sponge S/W Chocolate or Vanilla	,,	92	,,	323
Sponge Gateaux w/chocolate ..	,,	117	,,	413
Sponge Gateau w/Raspberry ..	,,	111	,,	391
Sponge S/W Jam Buttercream ..	,,	100	,,	353
Sultana & Bramley Apple ..	,,	80	,,	283

Food	Quantities	Calories	Quantities	Calories
Sultana Cut	1 oz	97	100 g	342
Swiss Roll				
Apricot	,,	102	,,	359
Blackcurrant ..	,,	100	,,	353
Chocolate Sponge ..	,,	116	,,	408
Coffee Sponge ..	,,	121	,,	425
Chocolate Swiss ..	,,	113	,,	397
Jam Swiss	,,	82	,,	290
Desserts & Pies)				
Apple Pie	1 oz	85	100 g	301
Apple Pies, individual ..	each	192	—	—
Apple Puffs, individual ..	,,	200	—	—
Apple Tarts, individual ..	,,	160	—	—
Baked Alaska	1 oz	75	100 g	266
Black Forest Gateau				
(frozen) ..	,,	79	,,	278
Cheesecake				
Blackcurrant ..	,,	75	,,	263
Cherry	,,	73	,,	258
Pineapple	,,	78	,,	275
Choc. Layer Cake (frozen)	,,	96	,,	340
Chocolate & Cherry				
Gateau (frozen) ..	,,	77	,,	272
Chocolate Nut Meringue ..	,,	85	,,	299
Danish & Apple ..	,,	89	,,	312
Danish Sultana ..	,,	108	,,	380
Gooseberry Slice ..	,,	72	,,	254
Lemon Cream Flan ..	,,	104	,,	365
Raspberry Meringue ..	,,	84	,,	297
Raspberry & Redcurrant				
Pies ..	each	182	—	—
Rhubarb Tart, large ..	,,	52	,,	185

Cakes, Pies, Cake Mixes, Pastries

Food	Quantities	Calories	Quantities	Calories
Strawberry Meringue	100 g	91	100 g	321
Waffles	,,	108	,,	380
(small cakes)				
Apricot Slices	each	251	—	—
Blackcurrant Sundaes	,,	204	—	—
Cakes w/Choc. Buttercream	,,	133	—	—
Chocolate Eclairs	,,	127	—	—
Chocolate Sponge Curls	,,	200	—	—
Chorley Cakes	,,	290	—	—
Corn Crisp	,,	130	—	—
Cream Puffs	,,	233	—	—
Creme Patisserie Doughnuts	,,	118	—	—
Custard Slices	,,	204	—	—
Doughnuts	,,	174	—	—
Eccles–all butter	,,	171	—	—
Egg Custard Tarts	,,	219	—	—
Fondant Fancies	,,	112	—	—
Meringues	,,	118	—	—
Rice Crisp	,,	92	—	—
Rum Baba	,,	210	—	—
Snowballs	,,	103	—	—
Sponge Curls, Blackcurrant	,,	188	—	—
Viennese–all butter	,,	283	—	—
MARY BAKER MIXES				
Baked Alaska	1 packet	990	—	—
Black Forest Gateau	,,	1485	—	—
Butterfly Tops	,,	830	—	—
Cherry Shortcake	,,	1383	—	—
Chocolate Sandwich	,,	1349	—	—
Chocolate Tops	,,	830	—	—
Fruit Cake	,,	1340	—	—

Food	Quantities	Calories	Quantities	Calories
Lemon Meringue Crunch ..	1 packet	1132	—	—
Lemon Tops	,,	830	—	—
Orange Tops	,,	831	—	—
Profiteroles	,,	936	—	—
Vanilla Sandwich ..	,,	1372	—	—
Yogurtcake, Apricot ..	,,	1081	—	—
Yogurtcake, Cherry & Almond ..	,,	1052	—	—
MR KIPLING				
All Butter Shorties ..	each	139	—	—
Almond Slice	,,	140	—	—
Apple Bakewell Tart ..	1 oz	105	100 g	369
Apple/Blackcurrant Pies ..	each	179	—	—
Apple Pies	,,	200	—	—
Apple Sundaes ..	,,	197	—	—
Bakewell Slices ..	,,	174	—	—
Bakewell Tart	1 oz	116	100 g	408
Blackcurrant Sundaes	each	195	—	—
Cherry Bakewell Tarts	,,	202	—	—
Cherry Slices	,,	148	—	—
Cherry Walnut Slices ..	,,	140	—	—
Chocolate Swiss Roll ..	1 oz	91	100 g	319
Coconut Macaroons ..	each	106	—	—
Coffee Gateau ..	1 oz	106	100 g	373
Country Slices ..	each	119	—	—
Fudge Brownies ..	,,	157	—	—
Jam Swiss Roll ..	1 oz	81	100 g	286
Jam Tarts	each	131	—	—
Mince Pies	,,	205	—	—
Olde English Fruit Pies	,,	151	—	—
Raspberry Bakewell ..	1 oz	104	100 g	368

Cakes, Pies, Cake Mixes, Pastries

Food	Quantities	Calories	Quantities	Calories
Raspberry/Redcurrant Pies	each	190	—	—
Treacle Tarts	1 oz	98	100 g	347
Viennese Splits	each	85	—	—
ROYAL MIXES				
Chocolate Orange Crunch	1 packet	690	—	—
Coffee Crunch	,,	694	—	—
Lemon Crunch	,,	818	—	
Original Cheesecake	,,	718	—	
VIOTA (mixes)				
(large cakes)				
Chocolate Fudge	1 packet	1400	100 g	368
Cornish Tea Sponge	,,	1224	(made-up)	347
Cornish Tea Sponge w/jam filling	,,	1464	,,	363
Golden Shred Orange Marmalade				
Madeira	,,	1553	,,	345
Malt Layer Cake	,,	1749	,,	399
Walnut Layer Cake	,,	1427	,,	413
(small cakes)				
Afternoon Tea Cakes	each	74	1 packet	1324
Carnival Cakes	,,	66	,,	1056
Chocolate Cup Cakes				
with water icing	,,	93	,,	934
with fudge icing	,,	144	,,	1437
Coconut Macaroons	,,	63	,,	754
Iced Fairy Cakes	,,	65	,,	1040
Lemon Cup Cakes				
with water icing	,,	99	,,	993
with fudge icing	,,	156	,,	1559
Orange Frosted Cakes	,,	66	,,	1059

Food		Quantities	Calories	Quantities	Calories
VIOTA 'ECONOMIXES'					
Baked Sponge Pudding	..	each	116	1 packet	696
Chocolate Sponge, filled		,,	107	,,	1070
Crumble	.. ..	,,	190	,,	1140
Ginger Cake	..	,,	98	,,	977
Rock Cakes w/currants		,,	106	,,	1271
Scones	.. ..	,,	82	,,	659
Shortbread	..	,,	156	,,	1249
Small Cakes	..	,,	56	,,	670
Small Cakes, iced	..	,,	69	,,	828
Sponge Cake, filled	..	,,	70	,,	696
Yorkshire Pudding	..	,,	116	,,	696
WAITROSE					
(large cakes)					
Angel	.. .. ..	1 oz	122	100 g	429
Battenburg	.. ..	,,	105	,,	370
Cherry Genoa	.. ..	,,	94	,,	331
Chocolate	.. ..	,,	141	,,	496
Chocolate Swiss Roll	..	,,	104	,,	366
Corn Crisp	.. ..	,,	145	,,	510
Country Style Fruit Cake		,,	104	,,	366
Date & Walnut	..	,,	88	,,	310
Dundee	.. ..	,,	88	,,	310
French Jam Sandwich		,,	102	,,	359
Jamaica Ginger	..	,,	91	,,	320
Jam Swiss Roll	..	,,	92	,,	324
Jam Vanilla Swiss Roll		,,	104	,,	366
Madeira	.. ..	,,	109	,,	384
Rice Crisp	.. ..	,,	157	,,	552
Sponge Bar	.. ..	,,	134	,,	472
Sponge Flan	.. ..	,,	56	,,	197

Cakes, Pies, Cake Mixes, Pastries

Food	Quantities	Calories	Quantities	Calories
Sponge Sandwich ..	1 oz	134	100 g	472
Sultana	,,	94	,,	331
Swiss Roll, chocolate covered	,,	124	,,	436
Swiss Roll, apricot ..	,,	90	,,	317
Swiss Roll, strawberry vanilla	,,	102	,,	359
Swiss Roll, chocolate vanilla	,,	100	,,	387
Trifle Sponge	,,	56	,,	197
Walnut Layer Cake ..	,,	121	,,	426
(small cakes)				
Almond Slices ..	,,	112	,,	387
Apple Pies	,,	54	,,	190
Blackcurrant Pies ..	,,	54	,,	190
Chocolate Cup Cakes	,,	195	,,	686
Eccles Cakes	,,	147	,,	517
Eclairs, Chocolate covered	,,	199	,,	700
Jam Tarts	,,	136	,,	475
Lemon Curd Tarts ..	,,	143	,,	503
Madelines	,,	70	,,	246
Meringues	,,	141	,,	496
Orange & Lemon Cup Cakes	,,	195	,,	686
Raspberry/Redcurrant Pies	,,	56	,,	197
Swiss Roll, chocolate covered	,,	103	,,	362
Swiss Roll, chocolate covered (buttercream)	,,	126	,,	443
SAFEWAY				
Cheesecake mix	1|oz	89	100 g	315
Cut Cherry Genoa ..	,,	90	,,	318

Food	Quantities	Calories	Quantities	Calories
Cut Dundee Cake ..	1 oz	89	100 g	312
Cut Sultana Cake ..	,,	102	,,	360
Shortcrust Pastry Mix	,,	141	,,	495
TESCO				
Apple & Jam Nut Dessert	1 oz	121	100 g	427
Chocolate Dessert ..	,,	128	,,	452
Chocolate Iced ..	,,	124	,,	438
Chocolate Gateau ..	,,	129	,,	456
Jaffa Dessert	,,	121	,,	428
Marble Cake	,,	124	,,	438
Meringue Nests ..	,,	105	,,	371
Mince Pies	,,	112	,,	394
'Rondo' Almond ..	,,	119	,,	420
'Rondo' Cherry ..	,,	124	,,	438
Sponge Fingers ..	,,	108	,,	382
Sponge Flan Case ..	,,	92	,,	323
Swiss Rolls				
Apricot Jam ..	,,	116	,,	408
Choc. filled	,,	116	,,	408
Choc. coated ..	,,	119	,,	418
Hazelnut	,,	121	,,	427
Iced Marzipan ..	,,	118	,,	416
Strawberry	,,	106	,,	374
Cake Decorations)				
Crunch Nut Topping ..	,,	141	—	—
100's & 1000's ..	,,	106	—	—
Jelly Diamonds ..	,,	102	—	—
Orange & Lemon Slices	,,	91	—	—
Sugar Strands, assorted	,,	105	—	—
Sugar Strands, chocolate	,,	119	—	—

Cakes, Pies, Cake Mixes, Pastries

Food	Quantities	Calories	Quantities	Calories
(Mixes)				
Batter	1 oz	141	100 g	495
Cheesecake	,,	84	,,	297
Choc. Sandwich	,,	128	,,	451
Crumble	,,	191	,,	671
Flaky Pastry	,,	164	,,	577
Luxury Sponge	,,	122	,,	431
Shortcrust Pastry	,,	142	,,	500
Sponge Sandwich	,,	194	,,	682
Tea Cakes, Iced	,,	106	,,	375

Cereals

In this new edition of *The Pocket Calorie Guide to Branded Foods* a new section has been made for Pasta and Rice products. This section is therefore only for breakfast-style cereals. Since the calorific content of some of the more popular types varies very little they have been listed under product, not brand-name as in the previous edition.

Food	Quantities	Calories	Quantities	Calories
Miscellaneous				
Bran Flakes	1 oz	100	100 g	352
Cornflakes	,,	100	,,	352
Porridge Oats	,,	110	,,	387
Swiss Style (muesli) ..	,,	105	,,	370
Wholewheat Biscuits ..	,,	100	,,	352
ALLINSON				
Bran Plus	1 oz	63	100 g	222
Broad Bran	,,	43	,,	142
Crunchy Bran	,,	63	,,	222
BEMAX	1 oz	85	100 g	300
BIRDS				
Grape Nuts	1 oz	100	100 g	352

Cereals

Food		Quantities	Calories	Quantities	Calories
HOLLAND & BARRETT					
Sugar Free Muesli	..	1 oz	106	100 g	372
JORDANS					
Original Crunchy	..	1 oz	120	100 g	424
KELLOGGS					
All Bran	.. ..	1 oz	70	100 g	247
Bran Buds	.. ..	,,	76	,,	268
Coco Pops	.. ..	,,	101	,,	357
Country Store	.. ..	,,	100	,,	353
Crunchy Nut Corn Flakes		,,	107	,,	377
Frosties	.. ..	,,	100	,,	355
Rice Krispies	.. ..	,,	99	,,	350
Ricicles	.. ..	,,	100	,,	353
Smacks	.. .. ..	,,	106	,,	372
Special K	.. ..	,,	83	,,	292
Sultana Bran	.. ..	,,	101	,,	355
Summer Orchard	..	,,	95	,,	334
LYONS					
Ready Brek–all flavours		1 oz	110	100 g	390
MEADOW FARM					
Toasted Bran	.. ..	1 oz	101	100 g	356
NABISCO					
Cubs	.. .. ..	1 oz	101	100 g	355
Shredded Wheat	..	1 biscuit	80	,,	355
Shreddies	.. ..	1 oz	105	,,	370
PREWETTS					
Golden Grains	..	1 oz	107	100 g	376

Food	Quantities	Calories	Quantities	Calories
Muesli, bran	1 oz	87	100 g	308
Muesli, de-luxe	,,	110	,,	388
Muesli, honey	,,	103	,,	364
Wholewheat Flakes	,,	101	,,	356
QUAKER				
Golden Oaties	1 oz	108	100 g	379
'Harvest Crunch'				
Bran & Apple	,,	129	,,	453
U.K.	,,	126	,,	445
Hot Bran Cereal	,,	92	,,	325
Oat Krunchies	,,	108	,,	381
Puffed Wheat	,,	106	,,	374
Sugar Puffs	,,	104	,,	367
WEETABIX				
Bran Fare	1 oz	65	100 g	228
Farmhouse Bran	,,	85	,,	300
Farmhouse Bran w/Banana				
& Apple	,,	95	,,	335
Farmhouse Bran w/Honey				
& Nuts	,,	95	,,	335
Weetaflake	,,	95	,,	335
Weetaflake 'n' Raisin	,,	95	,,	335

Crisps and Savoury Snacks

These can be insidious so count carefully—and do not make a habit of eating them!

Food	Quantities	Calories	Quantities	Calories
CRISPS (average, all brands)				
Plain, Salted, Salt & Vinegar	1 oz	135	100 g	476
Cheese & Onion ..	,,	150	,,	529
Other flavours (average)	,,	160	,,	564
BIRD'S EYE				
Brunchies	each	130	—	—
Cheesies	,,	60	—	—
Chicklets	,,	130	—	—
GOLDEN WONDER				
Country Crunch, bacon ..	1 oz	121	100 g	425
Ringos: Cheese & Onion ..	,,	124	,,	438
Ringos: Salt & Vinegar ..	,,	128	,,	451
Wotsits: Cheesy ..	,,	162	,,	571
HUNTLEY & PALMER				
Cheese Sticks	1 biscuit	22	—	—
Cheese & Celery Sticks ..	,,	22	—	—
Cheese & Tomato Sticks ..	,,	22	—	—

Food		Quantities	Calories	Quantities	Calories
INTERNATIONAL					
Cheesy Corn Curls	..	1 oz	128	100 g	454
Cheese & Ham Snips	..	,,	145	,,	511
Cheesy Puffs	.. ..	,,	145	,,	511
Cheese Savouries	..	,,	150	,,	527
Crispy Sticks	.. ..	,,	138	,,	487
Potato Rings & Sticks	..	,,	154	,,	533
Potato Scoops	.. ..	,,	170	,,	599
Streakies	.. ..	,,	129	,,	456
MARKS AND SPENCER					
Barbecue Sticks	..	1 oz	138	100 g	485
Bucctini	.. ..	,,	134	,,	472
Loops	.. .. ..	,,	136	,,	480
Potato Rings, Sticks, Thins		,,	145	,,	510
Prawn Cocktail Snacks	..	,,	138	,,	486
Salt & Vinegar Chiplets	..	,,	138	,,	486
Savoury Puffs	.. ..	,,	170	,,	600
Sizzles	.. .. ..	,,	129	,,	455
Wheat Crunchies	..	,,	137	,,	482
PEAK FREAN					
Cheeselets	.. ..	1 biscuit	3	—	—
Twiglets, large	..	,,	6	—	—
Twiglets, small	..	,,	3	—	—
PREWETTS					
Brazilian Mix	.. ..	1 oz	116	100 g	407
5-Cereal Savoury Mix	..	,,	116	,,	407
Rissole Mix	.. ..	,,	97	,,	341

Crisps and Savoury Snacks

Food	Quantities	Calories	Quantities	Calories
SAFEWAY				
Bacon Streaks	1 oz	129	100 g	455
Chicken Wattles	,,	125	,,	440
Onion Rings	,,	146	,,	516
Prawn Cocktail Wattles	,,	124	,,	438
Ready Salted Crunchy Sticks	,,	134	,,	472
Ready Salted Potato Sticks	,,	143	,,	505
Salt & Vinegar Crunch Sticks	,,	138	,,	487
Salt & Vinegar Twirls	,,	133	,,	468
Savoury Puffs	,,	170	,,	600
Savoury Twiglets	,,	114	,,	400
TESCO				
Bacon Bites & Puffs	1 oz	139	100 g	491
Cheese Puffs	,,	154	,,	541
Cheese & Onion Puffs	,,	145	,,	511
Corn Curls	,,	48	,,	170
Moons	,,	136	,,	480
Onion Rings	,,	37	,,	130
Potato Rings	,,	151	,,	533
Prawn Cocktail Snacks	,,	138	,,	487
Savoury Sticks	,,	121	,,	426
WAITROSE				
Potato Sticks	1 oz	156	100 g	549
Savoury Puffs	,,	150	,,	528

Dairy Products, Fats, Oils (including non-dairy substitutes)

Most of the information in this section has been arranged under food category rather than brand-name because the majority of products have the same calorific content, regardless of manufacturer. Also included in this new edition are some non-dairy substitutes available in health shops. Low calorie spreads have purposely been omitted as the calorie content is listed on the packet.

Food	Quantities	Calories	Quantities	Calories
DAIRY PRODUCTS				
Butter	1 oz	225	25 g	197
Cheese, cottage				
Natural (average, all brands)	4 oz	107–119	100 g	95–105
Cheddar & Onion	„	125–148	„	110–130
Chives	„	114–123	„	100–108
Onion & Peppers	„	102	„	90
Pineapple	„	96–114	„	85–100
Prawn Cocktail	„	131–148	„	115–130
Salmon & Cucumber	„	125–136	„	110–120

Dairy Products, Fats, Oils

Food			Quantities	Calories	Quantities	Calories
Cheese, hard (average, all brands)						
Caerphilly	..	..	1 oz	105	100 g	370
Cheddar	..	..	,,	120	,,	420
Cheshire	..	..	,,	110	,,	388
Danish Blue	..	..	,,	114	,,	400
Derby	..	..	,,	110	,,	388
Double Gloucester		..	,,	110	,,	388
Edam	..	..	,,	90	,,	320
Emmenthal	..	..	,,	105	,,	370
Gorgonzola	..	..	,,	112	,,	395
Gouda	..	..	,,	96	,,	340
Gruyere	..	..	,,	120	,,	420
Jarlsberg	..	..	,,	100	,,	350
Lancashire	..	..	,,	100	,,	350
Leicester	..	..	,,	110	,,	390
Parmesan	..	..	,,	120	,,	416
Port Salut	..	..	,,	90	,,	315
Smoked	..	..	,,	110	,,	390
St. Paulin	..	..	,,	85	,,	300
Stilton	..	..	,,	135	,,	480
Wensleydale	..	..	,,	110	,,	390
Cheese, processed						
Cheese spread (average, all brands)			1 oz	80–85	,,	280–300
KRAFT						
Cracker Barrel	..		1 oz	120	100 g	420
Pizzagrill	..	..	,,	85	,,	300

Food	Quantities	Calories	Quantities	Calories
Slices				
Cheddar and 'Singles'	1 oz	88	100 g	310
Cheshire	,,	97	,,	345
ST. IVEL				
Family Favourites ..	1 oz	80	100 g	280
Gold Spinner	,,	80	,,	280
SLINKY				
Low-cal Cheese Spread ..	1 oz	37	100 g	129
WAITROSE				
Canadian Spread and Full				
Processed	,,	106	,,	373
Cheese, soft				
Boursin	1 oz	115	100 g	404
Blue Brie	,,	123	,,	435
Brie	,,	85	,,	300
Camembert ..	,,	75	,,	265
Cream				
Philadelphia ..	,,	90	,,	317
Waitrose, plain ..	,,	232	,,	817
Waitrose, flavoured ..	,,	210	,,	740
Curd	,,	35	,,	123
Quark, low fat ..	,,	25	,,	88
Cream				
Canned	1 oz	70	100 g	245
Cornish/Devon ..	,,	153	,,	575
Double & Extra Thick ..	,,	128	,,	450
Half Cream	,,	38	,,	135

Dairy Products, Fats, Oils

Food	Quantities	Calories	Quantities	Calories
Single & UHT ..	1 oz	55	100 g	195
Sour	,,	54	,,	195
Whipped	,,	108	,,	380
Whipping & UHT ..	,,	105	,,	370
Lard & Cooking Fat (average)	1 oz	262	25 g	230
Margarine (average, soft and hard) ..	1 oz	206	25 g	182
Milk				
Buttermilk (average) ..	1 pint	220	½ litre	233
Condensed,				
full fat	1 oz	92	100 g	325
half fat	,,	76	,,	267
Dried, skimmed				
as sold	,,	98	,,	345
reconstituted ..	1 pint	200	½ litre	220
Evaporated	1 fl. oz	48	1 decilitre	169
Fresh,				
full cream	1 pint	380	½ litre	402
Jersey	,,	440	,,	465
Fresh, semi-skimmed ..	,,	295	,,	260
Goats	,,	403	,,	355
Spray-dried,				
as sold	1 oz	140	100 g	495
reconstituted ..	1 pint	282	½ litre	310
Non-Dairy Fats				
Creamed Coconut ..	1 oz	175	25 g	154
Nutter & Suenut ..	,,	256	,,	225

Food		Quantities	Calories	Quantities	Calories
Non-Dairy Substitutes					
Granogen, as sold	..	1 oz	130	25 g	115
Plamil, C soya milk concentrate)	..	1 fl. oz	29	1 decilitre	103
Soya Milk	.. ..	,,	14	,,	51
Soyvita, reconstituted	..	1 pint	368	½ litre	405
Average all other brands	..	1 tsp.	10	—	—
Oil					
Corn (average)	..	1 fl. oz	208	25 ml	200
Olive (average)	..	,,	252	,,	220
Sunflower and Safflower	..	,,	208	,,	200
Soya Bean	.. ..	,,	208	,,	200
Vegetable (average)	..	,,	255	,,	225
Suet (average)	.. ..	1 oz	250	100 g	882
Yoghurt					
EDENVALE					
Natural	.. ..	1 oz	20	100 g	70
Chocolate	.. ..	,,	27	,,	96
Average, all other flavours		,,	25	,,	90
'Munch Bunch'					
Chocolate	.. ..	,,	32	,,	112
Average, all other flavours	..	,,	29	,,	102
'Snack Packs'					
Country Harvest/Muesli	..		,,	50	,,
Fruit & Nut	.. ..	,,	56	,,	196
'Tropical', average, all flavours	..	,,	28	,,	100

Dairy Products, Fats, Oils

Food	Quantities	Calories	Quantities	Calories
CHAMBOURCY				
Natural	1 oz	14	100 g	50
Lemon Fruit Curd	,,	29	,,	101
Average, all other flavours	,,	23–25	,,	80–90
'Whole Milk'				
Apricot/Fruits of the Forest				
'Bonjour', all flavours	,,	22	,,	78
'Chambor'				
Raspberry & Blackberry	,,	39	,,	139
Tropical Fruits	,,	37	,,	131
MARKS AND SPENCER				
Apricot & Almond	1 oz	31	100 g	108
Muesli	,,	32	,,	112
Natural	,,	20	,,	69
Average, all other flavours	,,	25	,,	90
ST. IVEL				
Natural	1 oz	17	100 g	60
'Countess', average all				
flavours	,,	33	,,	117
'Country Prize', Muesli	,,	27	,,	96
'Prize'				
Fruit (average)	,,	22	,,	79
Hazelnut	,,	25	,,	96
SKI				
Hazelnut	1 oz	26	100 g	93
Honey & Almond	,,	28	,,	98
Average, all other flavours	,,	25	,,	87

Food	Quantities	Calories	Quantities	Calories
WAITROSE				
Natural	1 oz	16	100 g	56
Average, all other flavours	,,	27	,,	96
Yoghurt, Drinking				
AMBROSIA				
Yoghurt Juices, all flavours	1 fl. oz	17–21	1 decilitre	60–75

Desserts

There seem to be many more ready-to-serve desserts on the market than when the previous edition was published. It is hoped that this section is fairly complete—it is certainly complete enough for those with a sweet tooth to occasionally indulge themselves. It may also be noted that not all the products in this section are very high in calories. Others are extremely high, however, so be careful.

Food	Quantities	Calories	Quantities	Calories
AMBROSIA (canned)				
Creamed Milk Puddings				
(all flavours)	1 oz	27	100 g	95
Devon Custard	,,	29	,,	103
Traditional Rice Pudding	,,	30	,,	107
BATCHELOR 'Pack-a-Pie'				
Plum	1 oz	68	100 g	241
Redcurrant & Raspberry	,,	85	,,	299
All other flavours (average)	,,	73	,,	256
BIRD'S				
Angel Delight (made-up,				
all flavours)	1 oz	41	100 g	144

Food	Quantities	Calories	Quantities	Calories
Blancmange (made-up, all flavours)	1 oz	30	100 g	106
Custard Powder (made-up)	,,	30	,,	106
Custard,				
'ready to serve' ..	,,	29	,,	102
'whisk-and-serve' ..	,,	26	,,	91
Dream topping, regular & w/added cream ..	,,	56	,,	197
Instant Whip (made-up, all flavours)	,,	30	,,	106
Lemon Pie Filling (made-up)	,,	20	,,	\70
Luxury Trifle Mixes (made-up)				
Fruit & Cherry ..	,,	37	,,	130
Mocha Rum ..	,,	53	,,	187
Peaches & Brandy ..	,,	44	,,	155
Strawberry & Sherry ..	,,	31	,,	109
Regular Trifle Mix (all flavours) ..	,,	28	,,	100
BIRD'S EYE (Frozen)				
Arctic Circles	one	155	—	—
Arctic Gateau	1/5 of cake	100	—	—
Arctic Log	1/6 of cake	100	—	—
Arctic Roll (small) ..	1/6 of roll	75	—	—
'Tub Desserts'				
Chocolate Lovely Milk	one tub	220	—	—
Melba, peach ..	,,	130	—	—
Mousse, Chocolate & Strawberry ..	,,	110	—	—

Desserts

Food	Quantities	Calories	Quantities	Calories
Supermousse, Chocolate, Strawberry & Raspberry ..	one tub	110	—	—
Choc 'N' Nut ..	,,	150	—	—
Neapolitan ..	,,	155	—	—
Superwhip	,,	885	—	—
Trifle	,,	120	—	—
Value Ice Cream Roll	1/6 of roll	55	—	—
BROWN AND POLSON				
Blancmange, chocolate ..	1 pint sachet	136	—	—
Blancmange, other flavours	,,	125	—	—
Instant Custard ..	1 oz	111	—	—
CHAMBOURCY				
Chamby	1 oz	32	100 g	114
Cheesecake, Family Size				
Blackcurrant ..	,,	71	,,	252
Strawberry	,,	56	,,	198
Cheesecakes, Individual				
Blackcurrant ..	,,	73	,,	257
Strawberry & Tangy Lemon	,,	78	,,	275
Creme Desserts, Chocolate & Vanilla	,,	39	,,	137
Dalky a la Creme				
Chocolate	,,	37	,,	132
Strawberry	,,	34	,,	121
Flanby, caramel ..	,,	28	,,	100
Fruit Sundaes				
Cocktail	,,	31	,,	111
Tropical Fruit ..	,,	30	,,	106
Raspberry	,,	34	,,	119

Food	Quantities	Calories	Quantities	Calories
Strawberry Sundae				
Special	1 oz	34	100 g	119
Supreme Desserts				
Chocolate & Vanilla	,,	32	,,	112
Mint & Chocolate	,,	35	,,	125
Strawberry & Vanilla	,,	38	,,	135
Voila 'Topping'	,,	41	,,	146
CHIVERS				
Jelly Creams, chocolate	1 packet	270	—	—
Jelly Creams, other flavours	,,	275		
Table Jellies	,,	410	—	—
COLMANS 'Dessert Toppings'				
Caramel & Chocolate	1 oz	85	100 g	300
Fruit flavours	,,	79	,,	280
CROSSE & BLACKWELL				
'Dessert Toppings'				
Double Top	1 oz	50	100 g	178
Tip Top	,,	31	,,	110
Custard Powder	,,	93	—	—
EDENVALE				
Caramel Supreme	1 oz	39	100 g	139
Cheesecake	,,	68	,,	239
Chocolate Cream Dessert	,,	41	,,	143
Chocolate Fool	,,	62	,,	217
Chocolate Supreme	,,	39	,,	139
Chocolate & Blackcurrant				
Whip	,,	44	,,	155
Creme Caramel	,,	42	,,	148

Desserts

Food			Quantities	Calories	Quantities	Calories
Fresh Cream Dessert	..		1 oz	41	100 g	143
Fruit Fool	..	..	,,	68	,,	238
Mandarin & Lemon Whip			,,	39	,,	139
Raspberry Trifle	..		,,	44	,,	155
Strawberry Supreme	..		,,	33	,,	116
Strawberry Trifle	..		,,	50	,,	176
Syllabub	..	..	,,	80	,,	281
FINDUS (frozen)						
Country Apple Pie	..		1 oz	86	100 g	302
Dairy Cream Sponge	..		,,	101	,,	355
Double Mousse,						
Strawberry/Vanilla	..		,,	39	,,	137
Raspberry/Vanilla	..		,,	43	,,	152
Chocolate/Vanilla	..		,,	38	,,	133
Lemon Cream Pie	..		,,	101	,,	358
Ripple Mousse						
Chocolate	..	..	,,	50	,,	177
Raspberry	..	..	,,	48	,,	171
Strawberry	..	..	,,	48	,,	171
Waffles	..	..	,,	87	,,	306
GRANNY SMITHS						
Custard Mix	..	..	1 oz	109	100 g	384
HEINZ						
'Sponge Puddings'						
Chocolate	..	..	1 oz	89	100 g	316
Mixed Fruit	..	..	,,	87	,,	307
Raspberry	..	..	,,	80	,,	282
Strawberry	..	..	,,	81	,,	285
Treacle	..	..	,,	81	,,	285

Food		Quantities	Calories	Quantities	Calories
HP					
'Dessert Sauces'					
Chocolate	.. ..	1 oz	87	100 g	305
Raspberry	.. ..	,,	31	,,	110
Strawberry	.. ..	,,	48	,,	170
LIBBY'S					
Creamed Rice	.. ..	1 oz	25	100 g	89
LYONS MAID					
'Dessert Sauces'					
Butterscotch	..	1 oz	89	100 g	314
Chocolate	.. ..	,,	80	,,	283
Raspberry & Strawberry		,,	75	,,	265
MARKS AND SPENCER					
Apple Cream Dessert	..	1 oz	48	100 g	170
Baked Rice Dessert	..	,,	31	,,	109
Delights,					
Chocolate & Caramel	..	,,	39	,,	139
Strawberry	.. ..	,,	33	,,	116
Desserts,					
Caramel	.. ..	,,	38	,,	135
Chocolate	.. ..	,,	41	,,	144
Double Decker,					
Black Cherry	..	,,	35	,,	124
Apricot	.. ..	,,	35	,,	124
Fruit Trifle, individual	..	,,	45	,,	158
Fruit Trifle, large	..	,,	47	,,	165
Jaffa Orange Dessert	..	,,	32	,,	114
Peach Melba Dessert	..	,,	32	,,	114
Rice Dessert × 2	..	,,	51	,,	179

Desserts

Food	Quantities	Calories	Quantities	Calories
Royales, Mandarin & Raspberry	1 oz	39	100 g	135
Whips,				
Chocolate	,,	52	,,	185
Strawberry	,,	43	,,	151
RAYNER BURGESS				
Dessert Toppings, all flavours	1 oz	76	100 g	267
RICH'S				
Coffee Rich Liquid	½ oz	22	100 g	153
Whip Topping	1 fl. oz	20	,,	276
ROWNTREE CREAMOLA				
Instant Custard Mix (as sold)	1 oz	119	100 g	418
Rice Creamola	,,	101	,,	357
Steamed/Baked Pudding Mix (as sold)	,,	81	,,	286
Tablet Jelly, all flavours (as sold)	,,	78	,,	275
ROSS (frozen)				
Apple Pie	1 oz	63	100 g	230
Apple & Blackberry Pie	,,	63	,,	230
Creme Caramel	,,	28	,,	100
Cheesecake, average, all flavours	,,	65	,,	235
Dairy Cream Sponge	,,	82	,,	290
Devonshire Individual Trifles	,,	45	,,	160

Food	Quantities	Calories	Quantities	Calories
Gateaux,				
Black Forest	1 oz	88	100 g	310
Coffee Mandarin	,,	85	,,	300
Devon Cream	,,	91	,,	320
Mandarin Cream	,,	79	,,	280
Rich Choc-n-Orange	,,	105	,,	370
Rum & Raisin	,,	91	,,	320
Strawberry & Cream	,,	63	,,	230
Lighterbite, average, all flavours	,,	76	,,	268
Supervalue				
Choc and Orange	,,	77	,,	270
Hazelnut	,,	94	,,	330
Strawberry & Yoghurt	,,	57	,,	200
Lemon Torte	,,	71	,,	250
Pineapple Pavlova	,,	77	,,	270
Profiteroles Choux	,,	114	,,	400
Profiteroles Sauce	,,	96	,,	340
Rhum Baba	,,	68	,,	240
Strawberry Meringue	,,	91	,,	320
Suisse Delice	,,	45	,,	160
Individual Desserts				
Apple Crumble & Custard	1 dessert	230	—	—
Apple & Blackberry Pie & Custard	,,	160	—	—
Apple Pie and Custard	,,	170	—	—
Bakewell Tart & Custard	,,	240	—	—
Bread Pudding & Custard	,,	270	—	—
Chocolate Sponge & Sauce	,,	140	—	—
Ginger Sponge & Custard	,,	180	—	—
Gooseberry Pie & Custard	,,	180	—	—
Ground Rice & Nutmeg	,,	160	—	—

Desserts

Food	Quantities	Calories	Quantities	Calories
Jam Roly Poly & Custard	1 dessert	340	—	—
Lemon Meringue Pie ..	,,	190	—	—
Lemon Sponge and Sauce	,,	130	—	—
Mincemeat Pie and Custard	,,	230	—	—
Plum & Apple Pie & Custard	,,	150	—	—
Plum Pudding & Rum Sauce	,,	300	—	—
Rhubarb Crumble & Custard	,,	170	—	—
Rice Pudding	,,	150	—	—
Sultana Sponge & Custard	,,	190	—	—
Treacle Tart & Custard ..	,,	240	—	—
ROYAL				
Crystal Jellies, all flavours	1 oz	100	100 g	352
Lemon Pie Filling ..	,,	100	,,	352
Simply Topping ..	,,	163	,,	575
SAFEWAY				
Custard Powder (as sold) ..	1 oz	94	100 g	330
ST. IVEL				
Creme Caramel ..	1 oz	31	100 g	110
'Fresh Cream Desserts'				
Fruit	,,	42	,,	148
Chocolate	,,	44	,,	154
'Souffle'				
Fruit	,,	45	,,	160
Chocolate	,,	52	,,	185
Trifles (average) ..	,,	41	,,	144

Food			Quantities	Calories	Quantities	Calories
'Wizard Mousse'						
Fruit	..	..	1oz	51	100 g	180
Chocolate	..	..	,,	50	,,	175
TESCO						
Dairy Cream Sponge						
(frozen)	..	..	1 oz	50	100 g	176
'Delights' (Mixes)						
Chocolate	..	..	,,	44	,,	155
Other flavours		..	,,	38	,,	134
Fresh Cream Trifle (frozen)			,,	50	,,	176
Jellies						
Blackcherry	..	..	,,	17	,,	59
Lemon	..	..	,,	29	,,	101
Orange	..	..	,,	36	,,	126
Mousses, average		..	,,	50	,,	176
Toppings,						
Custard Powder		..	,,	66	,,	234
Dessert Topping		..	,,	90	,,	317
WAITROSE						
(canned)						
Creamed Macaroni &						
Tapioca	..	..	1 oz	37	100 g	130
Creamed Rice	..	..	,,	42	,,	148
Pie Fillings,						
Apple	..	..	,,	27	,,	95
Blackberry & Apple		..	,,	22	,,	77
Blackcurrant		..	,,	29	,,	102
Cherry	..	..	,,	28	,,	98

Desserts

Food	Quantities	Calories	Quantities	Calories
(fresh dairy)				
Mousse,				
Chocolate	1 oz	29	100 g	102
Orange & Lemon	,,	26	,,	91
Peach & Cream	,,	34	,,	120
Strawberry	,,	27	,,	95
Strawberry & Cream	,,	34	,,	120
(frozen)				
Mousses, average, all flavours	,,	43	,,	152
(packet)				
Jellies, all flavours	,,	73	,,	257
Milk Desserts, all flavours	,,	150	,,	528
YOUNGS				
Cheesecake, all flavours	,,	74	,,	260

Drinks—Hot and Cold

This section has been re-arranged for the new edition. In line with the rest of the book all low calorie drinks have been omitted as the dietary information is available on the bottle or can. Also when the calorific content of same-brand sparkling drinks is the same they have been included as 'average—all other flavours'. It is still suggested that you refer to Jane Colin's *Pocket Calorie Guide to Safe Slimming* for details of alcoholic drinks. Beware of fruit juices—they are high in calories and of less nutritional value than the fresh fruit itself. For fruit juices and sparkling drinks the calories have not been given per fluid ounce as it's doubtful if anybody would ever drink less than a decilitre ($3\frac{1}{2}$ fluid ounces) at a time.

Food	Quantities	Calories	Quantities	Calories
Fruit Juices/Squashes				
BIOTTA				
Beetroot	—	—	1 decilitre	40
Breuss	—	—	"	37
Carrot	—	—	"	35
BIRD'S EYE				
Florida Grapefruit (reconstituted)	—	—	1 decilitre	25

Drinks

Food	Quantities	Calories	Quantities	Calories
Florida Orange (reconstituted)	—	—	1 decilitre	32
COLMANS 'Whole Fruit Drinks' (undiluted)				
Lime	1 fl. oz	25	1 decilitre	90
All other flavours ..	,,	27	,,	95
CORONA Blackcurrant Flavour				
Cordial	1 fl. oz	34	1 decilitre	119
Grapefruit Drink w/Pineapple	,,	29	,,	101
Average, all other flavours	,,	25–28	,,	90–100
C-VIT Blackcurrant Health Drink (undiluted)	—	—	1 decilitre	210
FINDUS Orange Juice (concentrated)	1 fl. oz	38	1 decilitre	133
HEINZ				
Grapefruit Juice ..	—	—	1 decilitre	66
Orange	—	—	,,	46
Pineapple	—	—	,,	57
Tomato	—	—	,,	24
HI-FRUIT STILL FRUIT DRINKS				
Apple & Honey ..	1 fl. oz	14	1 decilitre	50
Caribbean Fruit Drink ..	,,	14	,,	50
Orange	,,	13	,,	45

Food	Quantities	Calories	Quantities	Calories
HUNTS				
Grapefruit Juice, sweetened	—	—	1 decilitre	62
Orange Juice, unsweetened	—	—	,,	42
Orange Juice, sweetened ..	—	—	,,	54
Tomato Juice Cocktail ..	—	—	,,	16
INTERNATIONAL				
Apple Juice	—	—	1 decilitre	38
Grapefruit Juice ..	—	—	,,	39
Lemon & Lime Drink ..	1 fl. oz	25	,,	88
Lime Juice	,,	28	,,	96
Orange Juice	—	—	,,	45
Orange, Lemon & Pineapple Drink ..	1 fl. oz	28	1 decilitre	98
Whole Lemon/Orange ..	,,	33	,,	117
KIA-ORA (undiluted)				
Lemon & Orange Drink ..	1 fl. oz	8	1 decilitre	28
Orange & Pineapple Drink	,,	14	,,	50
Lemon/Lime Drink ..	,,	28	,,	98
LIBBY				
Good Start	—	—	1 decilitre	35
Grapefruit Juice, sweetened	—	—	,,	38
Grapefruit Juice, unsweetened ..	—	—	,,	31
Grapefruit 'C', sweetened	—	—	,,	58
Grapefruit 'C', reduced calories ..	—	—	,,	30
Orange Juice, sweetened	—	—	,,	51
Orange Juice, unsweetened	—	—	,,	33
Orange 'C', sweetened ..	—	—	,,	51

Drinks

Food	Quantities	Calories	Quantities	Calories
Orange 'C', reduced calories	—	—	1 decilitre	31
Tomato Juice	—	—	,,	20
MARKS AND SPENCER *(canned)*				
Caribbean	—	—	1 decilitre	55
Jaffa Grapefruit & Orange	—	—	,,	40
Lemon & Lime	—	—	,,	35
Pineapple	—	—	,,	41
Sunfruit	—	—	,,	47
Texas Pink Grapefruit	—	—	,,	30
(frozen, diluted)				
Caribbean Drink	—	—	,,	55
Orange Juice	—	—	,,	40
LINDAVIA				
Grape Juice, red & white	—	—	1 decilitre	63
MARTLETT				
Apple Juice Concentrate (diluted)	—	—	1 decilitre	24
Natural Apple Juice	—	—	,,	40
PREWETT 'Tetra Packs'				
Apple	—	—	1 decilitre	47
Grapefruit	—	—	,,	31
Orange	—	—	,,	33
Red Grape	—	—	,,	66
QUOSH *(undiluted)*				
Strawberry Cordial	1 fl. oz	33	1 decilitre	118
Average, all other flavours	,,	27–28	,,	95–100

Food	Quantities	Calories	Quantities	Calories
RIBENA *(undiluted)*	1 fl. oz	83	1 decilitre	293
Ribena, Baby, all flavours	,,	90	,,	316
ROBINSON *(undiluted)*				
Barley Water, all flavours	1 fl. oz	30	1 decilitre	110
ROSE'S				
Lime Juice Cordial ..	1 fl. oz	7	1 decilitre	24
SCHWEPPES				
Grapefruit Juice ..	—	—	1 decilitre	60
Orange Juice, sweetened	—	—	,,	55
Orange & Pineapple Juices, unsweetened ..	—	—	,,	47
Tomato Juice Cocktail ..	—	—	,,	17
SCHWEPPES				
Blackcurrant Cordial ..	1 fl. oz	38	1 decilitre	135
Ginger Cordial (non-alcoholic) ..	,,	26	,,	91
Lemon Drink	,,	31	,,	108
Lime Flavour Cordial ..	,,	27	,,	97
Peppermint Cordial (non-alcoholic) ..	,,	29	,,	103
Orange Squash ..	,,	31	,,	111
SPAR				
Pure Apple	—	—	1 decilitre	48
Pure Grapefruit ..	—	—	,,	44
Pure Orange	—	—	,,	51

Drinks

Food	Quantities	Calories	Quantities	Calories
SQUEEZ				
Pure Orange Juice ..	—	—	1 decilitre	40
SUN CRUSH 2-FOLD (cups)				
Lemon	1 fl. oz	54	1 decilitre	192
Orange	,,	57	,,	201
WAITROSE				
Apple, Pure Juice ..	—	—	1 decilitre	39
Blackcurrant Drink ..	1 fl. oz	65	,,	229
Lemon Barley Water ..	,,	42	,,	148
Lemon Drink	,,	36	,,	127
Lemon & Lime Drink ..	,,	10	,,	35
Lemon Squash ..	,,	36	,,	127
Lime Juice Cordial ..	,,	32	,,	113
Orange Drink	,,	39	,,	137
Orange Juice	—	—	,,	21
Orange Squash ..	1 fl. oz	39	,,	137
Pineapple Juice ..	—	—	,,	46
Tomato Juice	—	—	,,	14
Hot Beverages				
Bovril	1 oz	49	1 teaspoon	12
Cocoa, unsweetened ..	,,	130	,,	20
Drinking Chocolate ..	,,	112	,,	28
Instant Hot Chocolate Mix	,,	115	,,	29
Malted Milk	,,	106	,,	26
Yeast Extract	,,	50	,,	13
Milk Shake Syrups & *Flavoured Milk*				
CRUSHA *(syrup)*				
Chocolate	1 oz	45	1 decilitre	160

Food	Quantities	Calories	Quantities	Calories
All other flavours	1 oz	31	1 decilitre	110
MARKS AND SPENCER				
Chocolate Flavoured Milk	—	—	,,	101
Strawberry Flavoured Milk	—	—	,,	75
RAYNER/BURGESS *(syrup)*				
Banana, Strawberry ..	1 oz	61	,,	214
Chocolate, Milk ..	,,	60	,,	212
Chocolate, Plain ..	,,	55	,,	194
Sparkling Drinks				
CARIBA	—	—	1 decilitre	35
COCA COLA	—	—	1 decilitre	40
CORONA				
Coola	—	—	1 decilitre	42
Ginger Beer	—	—	,,	29
Iron Brew	—	—	,,	45
Average, all other flavours	—	—	,,	20–25
CRESTA				
Blackcurrant & Strawberry	1 fl. oz	10	1 decilitre	35
Average, all other flavours	,,	8	,,	28
FANTA				
Lemonade & Limeade ..	—	—	1 decilitre	25
Orangeade & Sparkling Lemon ..	—	—	,,	35
Cream Soda, Ginger Beer & Raspberryade ..	—	—	,,	30

Drinks

Food		Quantities	Calories	Quantities	Calories
5-ALIVE					
Citrus and Tropical	..	—	—	1 decilitre	48
HI-C	.. .. ..	—	—	1 decilitre	45
HUNTS					
American Ginger Ale	..	—	—	1 decilitre	28
Bitter Lemon	.. ..	—	—	,,	34
Dry Ginger Ale	..	—	—	,,	16
Lemonade	.. ..	—	—	,,	24
Tonic	.. .. ..	—	—	,,	24
IDRIS					
American Ginger Ale	..	—	—	1 decilitre	28
Bitter Lemon	.. ..	—	—	,,	34
Ginger Beer	.. ..	—	—	,,	47
Shandy	.. .. ..	—	—	,,	25
Tonic	.. .. ..	—	—	,,	24
LILT	.. .. ..	—	—	1 decilitre	49
LUCOZADE	.. ..	—	—	1 decilitre	72
ORELIA					
Sparkling Orange Drink	..	—	—	1 decilitre	48
PEPSI COLA	.. ..	—	—	1 decilitre	46
RIBENA, sparkling	..	—	—	1 decilitre	62
SAFEWAY					
American Ginger Ale	..	—	—	1 decilitre	33

Food	Quantities	Calories	Quantities	Calories
Cherryade	—	—	1 decilitre	25
Cola	—	—	,,	37
Dry Ginger Ale ..	—	—	,,	22
Lemonade	—	—	,,	23
Limeade	—	—	,,	22
Orange	—	—	,,	30
SCHLOER				
Apple	—	—	1 decilitre	35
Grape	—	—	,,	49
SCHWEPPES				
American Ginger Ale ..	—	—	1 decilitre	36
Bitter Lemon	—	—	,,	32
Dry Ginger Ale ..	—	—	,,	15
Ginger Beer	—	—	,,	34
Lemonade	—	—	,,	29
Lemonade Shandy ..	—	—	,,	25
Orange	—	—	,,	43
Russchian	—	—	,,	23
Tonic	—	—	,,	20
SPAR				
American Ginger Ale ..	—	—	1 decilitre	34
Bitter Lemon	—	—	,,	43
Tonic	—	—	,,	33
SEVEN-UP	—	—	1 decilitre	39
TANGO				
Grapefruit	—	—	1 decilitre	45
Lemon & Lime ..	—	—	,,	37
Orange	—	—	,,	46

Drinks

Food		Quantities	Calories	Quantities	Calories
TOP DECK					
Lemonade Shandy	..	—	—	1 decilitre	25
Limeade & Lager	..	—	—	„	32
WAITROSE					
American Ginger Ale	..	—	—	1 decilitre	28
Apple Crush	.. ..	—	—	„	35
Bitter Lemon	.. ..	—	—	„	35
Blackcurrant Crush	..	—	—	„	35
Cola	.. .. ..	—	—	„	148
Dry Ginger Ale	..	—	—	„	28
Ginger Beer	.. ..	—	—	„	46
Lager & Lime	.. ..	—	—	„	32
Lemonade	.. ..	—	—	„	35
Lemonade Shandy	.. ..	—	—	„	25
Lemon & Lime	.. ..	—	—	„	35
Orange Drink	.. ..	—	—	„	35
Tonic Water	.. ..	—	—	„	28

Fish

Anybody on a slimming diet should try to eat plenty of fish which is full of goodness and, if not fried, very low in calories. There is such a large variety of ready-to-eat fish dishes available now, most of which are listed below. Fresh-frozen fish has not been included.

Food	Quantities	Calories	Quantities	Calories
BATCHELOR 'Vesta Meals'				
Paella	1 pkt (serves 2)	660	—	—
Prawn Curry	,,	709	—	—
BEJAM (*frozen*)				
Cod Steaks, breaded & fried	1 oz	49	100 g	173
Dolar Chips, fried	,,	48	,,	170
Kipper, 'boil in bag'	,,	48	,,	170
Plaice,				
stuffed w/mushroom,				
grilled	,,	52	,,	184
stuffed w/ham & cheese	,,	57	,,	200
stuffed w/prawns	,,	52	,,	184
Plaice, whole boneless &				
breaded	,,	48	,,	168
Scampi, fried	,,	68	,,	241

Fish

Food	Quantities	Calories	Quantities	Calories
BIRD'S EYE				
'Breaded Fish'				
Cod Fish Fingers .. one		45	—	—
Cod in Crisp Crunch Crumb .. ,,		185	—	—
Fish Cakes,				
Cod .. .. .. ,,		60	—	—
Salmon .. .. ,,		70	—	—
Savoury .. .. ,,		65	—	—
Haddock in Crisp Crunch Crumb ,,		185	—	—
Plaice in Crisp Crunch				
Crumb .. ,,		65	—	—
Value Fish Fingers .. ,,		45	—	—
'Fish in Batter'				
Crispy Cod Fingers .. ,,		55	—	—
Crispy Cod Fries .. 7 oz pkt		350	—	—
Crispy Cod Steaks .. one		175	—	—
Crispy Haddock Steaks .. ,,		175	—	—
Crispy Plaice Fillets .. 1 oz		60	100 g	211
Crispy Plaice, Whole .. ,,		55	,,	194
Oven Crispy Cod Steaks .. one		230	—	—
Oven Crispy Cod Fish				
Fingers .. ,,		80	—	—
Oven Crispy Fish 'n' Chips 1 pkt		470	—	—
Oven Crispy Haddock				
Steaks .. one		230	—	—
'MenuMaster Fish in Sauce'				
Cod in Butter .. .. 1 pkt		160	—	—
Cod in Cheese .. ,,		175	—	—
Cod in Mushroom .. ,,		180	—	—
Cod in Parsley .. ,,		150	—	—
Cod in Shrimp Flavour .. ,,		165	—	—
Plaice in Cream .. ,,		140	—	—

Food	Quantities	Calories	Quantities	Calories
Smoked Cod in Butter	,,	160	—	—
Captain's Pie	8 oz	270	—	—
Battercrisp Cod Portions	1 oz	55	100 g	193
Battercrisp Haddock Portions	,,	64	,,	224
Battered Cod Steaks	,,	49	,,	173
Battered Haddock Steaks	,,	45	,,	158
Cod Steak in Breadcrumbs	,,	30	,,	105
Cod Fillets in Breadcrumbs	,,	31	,,	110
Cod Steak in Butter Sauce	,,	23	,,	81
Cod Steak in Parsley Sauce	,,	19	,,	65
Cod Steak in Cheese Sauce	,,	26	,,	89
Cod Steak in Seafood Sauce	,,	20	,,	71
Economy Fish Fingers	,,	51	,,	180
Fish Cakes	,,	33	,,	118
Fish Portion in Breadcrumbs	,,	30	,,	105
Fish Steak in Butter Sauce	,,	25	,,	87
Fish Steak in Parsley Sauce	,,	20	,,	72
Haddock Fillets in Breadcrumbs	,,	31	,,	110
Haddock Fish Fingers	,,	54	,,	189
Haddock in Breadcrumbs	,,	30	,,	107
Hake Steak in Breadcrumbs	,,	30	,,	107
Kipper Fillets with Butter	,,	54	,,	191
Plaice Fillets in Breadcrumbs	,,	37	,,	131
Plaice, Whole in Breadcrumbs	,,	33	,,	116
Smoked Haddock with Butter	,,	29	,,	101

Fish

Food	Quantities	Calories	Quantities	Calories
'New From France'				
Coquilles	1 oz	33	100 g	115
Fish Gratin	,,	52	,,	183
INTERNATIONAL *(frozen)*				
All Cod Fish Fingers ..	1 oz	49	100 g	172
Value Cod Fish Fingers ..	,,	52	,,	184
LIBBY *(canned)*				
Mackerel Fillets ..	1 oz	49	100 g	174
MARKS AND SPENCER				
Cod in Parsley Sauce ..	1 oz	27	100 g	94
Cod and Prawn Pie ..	,,	47	,,	165
Fish Cakes	,,	28	,,	100
Fish Casserole ..	,,	23	,,	82
Fish Fingers	,,	48	,,	168
Fish Souffles	,,	37	,,	129
Fisherman Pie	,,	39	,,	136
Kedgeree	,,	43	,,	150
Ocean Pie	,,	30	,,	107
Plaice, rolled	,,	33	,,	117
Plaice, stuffed				
Mushroom & Cheese ..	,,	34	,,	120
Prawn & Mushroom ..	,,	31	,,	109
Sea Food Pasta ..	,,	34	,,	121
Smoked Haddock Pie ..	,,	26	,,	92
Smoked Mackerel ..	,,	43	,,	150
Smoked Salmon ..	,,	40	,,	142
PRINCES *(canned)*				
Crab, drained	1 oz	25	100 g	88

Food	Quantities	Calories	Quantities	Calories
Kipper Fillets in Oil ..	1 oz	85	100 g	298
Mackerel in Oil ..	,,	62	,,	220
Mackerel in Tomato ..	,,	46	,,	161
Pilchards in Tomato Sauce	,,	36	,,	126
Prawns, drained ..	,,	27	,,	94
Salmon, pink & red ..	,,	44	,,	155
Sardines in Oil ..	,,	95	,,	334
Sardines in Tomato ..	,,	50	,,	177
Shrimps, drained ..	,,	27	,,	94
Tuna in Oil	,,	82	,,	290

ROSS *(frozen)*

Food	Quantities	Calories	Quantities	Calories
Battered,				
Crispy Cod	1 oz	48	100 g	170
Jumbo Cod Fingers ..	,,	48	,,	170
Oven Cod	,,	57	,,	200
Breaded, average all fish ..	,,	34	,,	120
Chunky Cod Pie ..	,,	43	,,	150
Cod Bake	,,	34	,,	120
Cod Crumble	,,	51	,,	180
Cod Steaks	,,	23	,,	80
Fish Cakes	,,	31	,,	110
Fish Fingers	,,	51	,,	180
Fish in Butter Sauce ..	,,	23	,,	80
Fish in Parsley Sauce ..	,,	17	,,	60
Kipper Fillets	,,	54	,,	190
Kipper Fillets with Butter	,,	57	,,	200
Kippered Mackerel Fillets	,,	60	,,	210
Smoked Haddock Fillets	,,	23	,,	80
Smoked Haddock Fillets				
with Butter	,,	25	,,	90

Fish

Food	Quantities	Calories	Quantities	Calories
Smoked Mackerel Fillets ..	1 oz	77	100 g	270
Smoked Whiting Fillets ..	,,	23	,,	80
SAFEWAY *(frozen)*				
Cod in Batter	1 oz	57	100 g	200
Cod in Breadcrumbs ..	,,	35	,,	125
Cod in Butter or Parsley Sauce	,,	23	,,	80
Fish Cakes	,,	31	,,	110
Fish Fingers & Cod Fish Fingers	,,	51	,,	180
Haddock in Batter ..	,,	57	,,	200
Haddock in Breadcrumbs ..	,,	35	,,	125
Haddock Fillets ..	,,	24	,,	85
Plaice in Breadcrumbs ..	,,	47	,,	165
TESCO *(canned)*				
Sild in Tomato Sauce ..	1 oz	58	100 g	203
Tuna	,,	80	,,	283
(frozen)				
Cod w/breadcrumbs ..	,,	30	,,	107
Cod w/butter sauce ..	,,	21	,,	73
Cod w/Parsley sauce ..	,,	19	,,	68
Fish Cakes	,,	31	,,	109
Fish Fingers	,,	56	,,	199
Prawns	,,	23	,,	80
Steaks/Batter	,,	57	,,	200
WAITROSE *(canned)*				
Red Salmon	1 oz	39	100 g	137
Tuna Fish	,,	53	,,	186

Food		Quantities	Calories	Quantities	Calories
(frozen)					
Baked Herrings	..	1 oz	54	100 g	190
Fish Cakes	.. ..	,,	61	,,	215
Fried Cod	.. ..	,,	40	,,	141
Fried Haddock	..	,,	50	,,	176
Fried Plaice	.. ..	,,	40	,,	141
Kipper Fillets	.. ..	,,	57	,,	201
Kippers	..	,,	31	,,	109
Plaice Fillets, smoked	..	,,	26	,,	91
Smoked Haddock Fillets	..	,,	28	,,	98
YOUNG'S *(frozen)*					
Battercrisp Cod/Haddock	..	1 oz	57	100 g	200
Buttered Kipper Fillets	..	1 pack	320	,,	190
Buttered Smoked Haddock	..	,,	230	,,	82
Fillets, Cod, Haddock, Plaice	..	1 oz	26	,,	92
Fish Fingers, Cod	..	each	50	—	—
Fish Pie	..	1 pack	290	100 g	145
Golden Seafood Platter w/sauce	..	,,	620	,,	354
Golden Scampi	..	,,	235	,,	207
Plaice Fillets, breaded	..	1 oz	40	,,	140
Potted Shrimps	..	1 pot	125	,,	250
Prawn Cocktail	..	1 pack	210	,,	168
Prawn Curry	..	,,	130	,,	74
Prawns, peeled	..	1 oz	34	,,	120
Salmon & Mushroom Supreme	..	1 pack	245	,,	175
Smoked Mackerel	..	,,	480	,,	240
Snails	.. .. ..	,,	272	,,	355
Sole & Asparagus Royale	..	,,	245	,,	120

Fruit

It is often erroneously thought that you may eat as much fruit as you like when dieting. This is not true as even fresh fruit contains a great deal of sugar and, of course, canned and bottled fruit is usually in syrup. It is preferable, therefore, to eat canned fruit which has been drained, or fruit that is canned in its own juice which is readily available. Unfortunately the figures supplied by the manufacturers were for undrained fruit so these are the figures shown below. You may safely reduce the number of calories to half if the fruit is well-drained. This does not, of course, apply to dried fruit! The calories per ounce for canned fruit have not been given as nobody is likely to eat less than $3\frac{1}{2}$ ounces (100 g) of canned fruit.

Food			Quantities	Calories	Quantities	Calories
BAXTERS (*canned & undrained*)						
All types	..	..	—	—	100 g	86
HARTLEYS (*canned & undrained*)						
Blackcurrants	..	..	—	—	,,	85
Damsons	..	..	—	—	,,	95
Gooseberries	..	..	—	—	,,	80

Food	Quantities	Calories	Quantities	Calories
Prunes	—	—	100 g	125
Raspberries	—	,,	,,	85
Rhubarb	—	—	,,	60
Strawberries	—	—	,,	115
INTERNATIONAL *(canned)*				
Pie Fillings, average ..	—	—	100 g	66
Prunes	—	—	,,	117
Raspberries	—	—	,,	85
Rhubarb	—	—	,,	60
Strawberries	—	—	,,	229
(dried)				
Glace Cherries ..	1 oz	60	,,	212
Prunes, no soak ..	,,	33	,,	116
Others, average ..	,,	70	,,	246
LIBBY *(canned)*				
Apple Barrel	—	—	100 g	40
Apricots	—	—	,,	69
Fruit Cocktail	—	—	,,	79
Grapefruit segments ..	—	—	,,	30
Mandarin Oranges ..	—	—	,,	56
Peaches	—	—	,,	69
Pear Halves	—	—	,,	69
Pineapple slices & tidbits ..	—	—	,,	57
PRINCES *(canned)*				
Apricots	—	—	100 g	106
Fruit Cocktail	—	—	,,	70
Fruit Salad	—	—	,,	95
Grapefruit	—	—	,,	60
Mandarin Oranges ..	—	—	,,	56

Fruit

Food	Quantities	Calories	Quantities	Calories
Peaches & Pears	—	—	100 g	77
Pineapple	—	—	,,	87
SAFEWAY *(canned)*				
Fast Pints	1 oz	139	100 g	490
Glace Cherries	,,	60	,,	212
(dried)				
Currant	,,	69	,,	243
Mixed Fruit	,,	69–71	,,	243–250
Seedless Raisin	,,	70	,,	246
Sultanas	,,	71	,,	250
TESCO *(dried)*				
Dates, sugar rolled	1 oz	77	100 g	273
Exotic Fruit & Nut	,,	79	,,	280
Prunes	,,	35	,,	122
Others, average	,,	70	,,	246
Pie Fillings *(canned)*				
Apple	—	—	,,	64
Apple & Blackberry	—	—	,,	92
Apple & Raspberry	—	—	,,	66
Apricot	—	—	,,	82
Cherry	—	—	,,	124
Gooseberry	—	—	,,	95
Strawberry	—	—	,,	84
WAITROSE				
Apricots in Apple Juice	—	—	100 g	37
Fruit Cocktail in Apple Juice	—	—	,,	39
Grapefruit in Natural Juice	—	—	,,	39

Food	Quantities	Calories	Quantities	Calories
Mandarins in Natural Juice	—	—	100 g	39
Peaches in Apple Juice ..	—	—	,,	39
Pears in Natural Juice ..	—	—	,,	37
Pineapples in Natural Juice ..	—	—	,,	45

Health Food Snacks

This section is new to this edition and should prove useful as so-called 'Health Foods' are now readily available in most parts of the country. Although some are high in calories they definitely supply more nutritional needs than sweets or cakes. If you feel the need for a little self-indulgence try to eat something from this section.

Food	Quantities	Calories	Quantities	Calories
ALLINSON				
Carob Coated Crunchy Bar	1 bar	151	—	—
Carob Coated Sesame Crunch	,,	105	—	—
Sesame Crunch	,,	188		
Wheateats, all flavours	,,	89	—	—
BELLIS				
Almond & Honey	1 bar	175	—	—
Apricot	,,	166	—	—
Fruit & Nut	,,	168	—	—
Sesame	,,	148	—	—
GRANOSE				
Apricot & Date	1 bar	86	—	—
Carob Fruit	,,	144	—	—

Food		Quantities	Calories	Quantities	Calories
Ginger & Pear	..	1 bar	116	—	—
Muesli & Pineapple	..	,,	125	—	—
HOLLYMILL					
Crunchy Slice	.. ..	1 bar	187	—	—
Fruit & Nut	.. ..	,,	175	—	—
Muesli	.. .. ..	,,	216	—	—
Protein	.. .. ..	,,	183	—	—
KALIBU 'Carob Bars'					
Crunch	.. .. ..	1 bar	375	—	—
Hazelnut	.. ..	,,	381	—	—
Mint	.. .. ..	,,	313	—	—
Nut & Raisin	.. ..	,,	340	—	—
Orange	.. .. ..	,,	313	—	—
Plain	.. .. ..	,,	313	—	—
KALIBU 'Carob Coated Bars'					
Molasses	.. ..	1 bar	139	—	—
Muesli Nut	.. ..	,,	145	—	—
ONLY NATURAL					
Sesame Snacks	..	1 bar	180	—	—
PREWETTS 'Fruit Bars'					
Banana	.. ..	1 bar	76	—	—
Date/Apple Dessert	..	,,	97	—	—
Date/Fig Dessert	..	,,	109	—	—
Fruit & Nut	.. ..	,,	85	—	—
Fruit/Nut Dessert	..	,,	129	—	—
Muesli Fruit	.. ..	,,	127	—	—

Health Food Snacks

Food	Quantities	Calories	Quantities	Calories
QUAKER				
'Harvest Crunch Bars'				
Almond	1 bar	80	—	—
Almond & Honey	1 oz	128	100 g	450
Peanut	1 bar	80	100 g	450
SHEPHERD BOY				
Apple, Fruit & Nut	1 bar	150	—	—
Banana, Fruit & Nut	,,	150	—	—
Sunflower Fruit & Nut	,,	188	—	—
SUNRISE				
Fruit Honey & Muesli Bars	1 bar	146	—	—

Ice Cream

Ice cream is not as high in calories as you might expect and, taken in moderation, it does relieve the monotony of a diet. However, don't forget that most of the more exotic types of ice cream (e.g. maple walnut, rum 'n' raisin) have many more calories than the average English ice cream. Happily it has been possible to include some of the more unusual types in this new edition.

Food		Quantities	Calories	Quantities	Calories
LYON'S MAID					
'Cutting Bricks'					
Black Cherry Ripple	..	1 brick	909	—	—
Chocolate Ripple	..	,,	925	—	—
Cornish Dairy	..	,,	903	—	—
Neapolitan	..	,,	834	—	—
Peach Melba	..	,,	925	—	—
Weight Watchers	..	,,	527	—	—
Vanilla	..	,,	846	—	—
'Family Bricks'					
Black Cherry Ripple	..	1 brick	432	—	—
Chocolate/Banana	..	,,	401	—	—
Cornish Dairy	..	,,	428	—	—
Neapolitan Gaiety	..	,,	397	—	—
Raspberry Ripple	..	,,	432	—	—
Toffee Ripple	..	,,	429	—	—
Vanilla	..	,,	402	—	—

Ice Cream

Food	Quantities	Calories	Quantities	Calories
'Gold Seal', 1 portion				
Black Cherry	100 ml	119	—	—
Caramel Toffee	,,	113	—	—
Coffee Hazelnut	,,	105	—	—
Chocolate Almond	,,	139	—	—
Mint Chocolate Chip	,,	105	—	—
Raspberry Peach Sundae	,,	105	—	—
'Handy Pack'				
Raspberry Ripple	1 pack	297	—	—
Vanilla	,,	261	—	—
'Individual Line'				
Bubble Ball	each	101	—	—
Caramel Fudge	,,	168	—	—
Chipwich (inc. biscuit)	,,	343	—	—
Choc/Banana Lolly (M/pack)	,,	46	—	—
Choc. Mint	,,	168	—	—
Cider Quench	,,	34	—	—
Coconut Flake	,,	172	—	—
Cola Quench	,,	38	—	—
Cornish Chocolate Sundae	,,	133	—	—
Cornish Raspberry Sundae	,,	97	—	—
Cornish Vanilla Choc. Ice	,,	126	—	—
Cornish Vanilla Kup	,,	110	—	—
Dark Satin Choc. Ice	,,	128	—	—
Fab	,,	73	—	—
Golden Orange	,,	57	—	—
Gold Seal Choc. Nut Sundae	,,	94	—	—
Gold Seal Mint Choc. Sundae	,,	91	—	—
Gold Seal Raspberry Sundae	,,	77	—	—

Food		Quantities	Calories	Quantities	Calories
Juice Bar, Grapefruit	..	each	45	—	—
Juice Bar, Orange & Pineapple	.. ..	,,	47	—	—
King Cone,					
Chocolate	.. ..	,,	219	—	—
Cornish Dairy	..	,,	208	—	—
Mint Chocolate	..	,,	202	—	—
Strawberry	.. ..	,,	191	—	—
Vanilla	.. ..	,,	203	—	—
Merlins Brew	.. ..	,,	65	—	—
Mini Bricks (M/Pack)	..	,,	57	—	—
Mr. Men (all flavours)	..	,,	25	—	—
Orange Maid	.. ..	,,	49	—	—
Real Milk Ice	.. ..	,,	50	—	—
Rock around the Choc	..	,,	129	—	—
Rocket (M/Pack)	.. ..	,,	29	—	—
Sherbet Monsters	..	,,	48	—	—
Silky Smooth Choc Ice	..	,,	132	—	—
Skull	.. .. ..	,,	80	—	—
Strawberry Mivvi	..	,,	78	—	—
Toffee Crumble	..	,,	180	—	—
Twin Lolly (M/Pack)	..	,,	37	—	—
Vanilla Bar	.. ..	,,	72	—	—
Van. Choc. Stick (M/Pack)		,,	136	—	—
Vanilla Kup	.. ..	,,	84	—	—
Zoom	.. .. ..	,,	44	—	—

MARKS AND SPENCER
'American Style'

Food		Quantities	Calories	Quantities	Calories
Chocolate Chip	..	1 oz	75	100 g	263
Toffee Almond	..	,,	64	,,	225

Ice Cream

Food	Quantities	Calories	Quantities	Calories
'Non Dairy'				
Neapolitan	1 oz	50	100 g	177
Vanilla	,,	49	,,	172
ROSS				
Chocolate & Chocolate Ripple . .	1 oz	51	100 g	180
Dairy Cornish	,,	45	,,	160
Neapolitan	,,	51	,,	180
Raspberry Ripple . .	,,	48	,,	170
'Soft Serve' (all flavours) . .	,,	51	,,	180
Strawberry . .	,,	48	,,	170
Strawberry & Vanilla . .	,,	54	,,	190
Vanilla	,,	48	,,	170
Vanilla Choc. Ice . .	,,	82	,,	290
SAFEWAY				
Chocolate Soft-Scoop . .	1 oz	51	100 g	180
Cornish	,,	48	,,	171
Raspberry Ripple . .	,,	46	,,	164
Raspberry Ripple Soft-Scoop . .	,,	51	,,	180
Vanilla	,,	52	,,	182
Vanilla Soft-Scoop . .	,,	51	,,	180
TESCO				
Choc. Ices	1 oz	43	100 g	150
'Easy Scoop', all flavours . .	,,	48	,,	170
Sorbet, Lemon & Orange . .	,,	25	,,	90
Vanilla	,,	60	,,	212

Food	Quantities	Calories	Quantities	Calories
WAITROSE				
'Continentale Dairy',				
Black Cherry	1 oz	53	100 g	186
Caramel Toffee ..	,,	57	,,	201
Chocolate Chip/Mint Choc				
Chip ..	,,	66	,,	232
Dairy Choc 'N' Nut Cones ..	each	273	—	—
Ice Cream Roll ..	1/6	59	1 roll	354
'Soft Scoop',				
Chocolate	1 oz	51	100 g	179
Neapolitan	,,	52	,,	183
WALLS (individual)				
Big Dipper,				
Strawberry	each	110	—	—
Vanilla	,,	110	—	—
Big Feast	,,	232	—	—
Choc. Bar,				
Dark & Golden ..	,,	130	—	—
Double Chocolate ..	,,	160	—	—
Golden Vanilla ..	,,	130	—	—
Midnight Mint ..	,,	140	—	—
Dracula	,,	50	—	—
Fame	,,	125	—	—
Cornetto,				
Choc & Nut ..	,,	195	—	—
Mint Choc Chip ..	,,	220	—	—
Raspberry Crush ..	,,	175	—	—
Rum & Raisin ..	,,	195	—	—
Strawberry	,,	185	—	—
Cup Italiano,				
Choc & Nut ..	,,	170	—	—

Ice Cream

Food	Quantities	Calories	Quantities	Calories
Passion Fruit Cocktail ..	each	110	—	—
Raspberry Crush ..	”	120	—	—
Strawberry	”	125	—	—
Funny Faces	”	75	—	—
Funny Feet	”	85	—	—
Individual Slices,				
Strawberry	”	60	—	—
Vanilla	”	65	—	—
Ice Cream Bar,				
Cornish	”	90	—	—
Golden Vanilla ..	”	85	—	—
'K9'	”	50	—	—
Mini Choc	”	45	—	—
Mini Fruit	”	30	—	—
Mini Milk, Strawberry &				
Vanilla	”	35	—	—
Orange Fruitie ..	”	60	—	—
Pineapple Split ..	”	90	—	—
Screwball (2 ball) ..	”	115	—	—
Sparkles,				
Orangeade	”	39	—	—
all other flavours ..	”	30	—	—
Starship 4	”	35	—	—
Strawberry Split ..	”	80	—	—
Tom & Jerry	each	50	—	—
Tub, Golden Vanilla ..	”	105	—	—
Woppas	”	40	—	—
(Family Size)				
Golden Vanilla	100 ml	87	—	—
'Italiano',				
Choc & Nut Capri ..	each	115	—	—
Mint Choc Croccante ..	”	122	—	—

Food	Quantities	Calories	Quantities	Calories
Toffee Fudge, Caramello	each	112	—	—
Tutti Frutti, Classico ..	,,	107	—	—
Raspberry Ripple ..	,,	105	—	—
Strawberry Ripple Slice ..	,,	102	—	—
Average, all other flavours	,,	90–100	—	—

Jam, Honey, Marmalade, Peanut Butter, Syrup

As the calorific value of different flavoured jams, marmalades, honey and syrups varies so slightly, the average for each brand has been taken. However the 'Whole Earth' jam sold in Health Food Stores has a lower calorie content as can be seen below. Savoury Pastes and Spreads are now in a separate section.

Food			*Quantities*	*Calories*	*Quantities*	*Calories*
Honey (average)	..	..	1 oz	90	100 g	320
Jam (average)	..	..	,,	75	,,	270
Jam, 'Whole Earth'		..	,,	33	,,	116
Lemon Curd/Cheese						
CHIVERS	..	..	,,	81	,,	285
COLMAN	..	..	,,	82	,,	290
HARTLEY	..	..	,,	84	,,	295
MOORHOUSE	..	..	,,	83	,,	293
SAFEWAY	..	..	,,	86	,,	303
SPAR	..	..	,,	80	,,	282
TESCO	..	..	,,	94	,,	331
WAITROSE	..	..	,,	86	,,	303
Marmalade (average)		..	,,	75	,,	265

Food	Quantities	Calories	Quantities	Calories
Marmalade, 'Whole Earth' ..	1 oz	33	100 g	116
Mincemeat				
HARTLEY	,,	84	,,	295
INTERNATIONAL ..	,,	73	,,	259
ROBERTSONS	,,	76	,,	268
SPAR	,,	67	—	236
WAITROSE	,,	37	,,	130
Peanut Butter				
GALES	,,	170	,,	600
HARMONY	,,	165	,,	582
INTERNATIONAL ..	,,	175	,,	616
PREWETT	,,	176	,,	620
SUN PAT	,,	177	,,	623
TESCO	,,	175	,,	616
Spread				
CADBURY'S Chocolate ..	,,	90	,,	320
Syrups (average) ..	,,	90	,,	320
Treacle, black	,,	80	,,	282

Meats, Savoury Pies and Ready-prepared Meals

The choice of available foods in this section has grown so enormously in the last few years that it has not been possible to include them all. However, there should be enough to choose from those listed here. Obviously, it is better for somebody who is trying to lose a lot of weight to stick to fresh grilled meat but, with the help of the following section, it should be possible for you to enjoy some ready-prepared meals.

Food	Quantities	Calories	Quantities	Calories
BATCHELOR				
'Canned Meats'				
Beef & Gravy	1 can	495	—	—
Beef & Kidney ..	,,	392	—	—
Beef & Onion	,,	508	—	—
Minced Beef & Onion ..	,,	467	—	—
'Snackpots'				
Beef Chow Mein ..	1 pot	205	—	—
Beef Risotto	,,	201	—	—
Chicken Supreme ..	,,	241	—	—
Curry & Rice with Beef ..	,,	230	—	—
Curry & Rice with Chicken	,,	246	—	—

Food		Quantities	Calories	Quantities	Calories
Sweet & Sour Chicken	..	1 pot	251	—	—
'Vesta Meals'					
Beef Risotto	.. ..	2 servings	635	—	—
Chicken Supreme	..	„	975	—	—
Chili con Carne	..	„	847	—	—
Chop Suey	.. ..	„	956	—	—
Chow Mein	.. ..	„	629	—	—
Curry & Rice w/Beef	..	„	963	—	—
Curry & Rice w/Chicken	..	„	822	—	—
Hot Beef Curry	..	„	901	—	—
Tacos	.. .. ..	„	503	—	—
Tostadas	.. ..	„	489	—	—
Vegetable Curry	..	„	791	—	—
BAXTER					
Scottish Haggis	..	1 oz	48	100 g	170
Scotch Mince	.. ..	„	31	„	110
BEANFEAST					
Bolognese	.. ..	1 oz	83	100 g	291
Chicken Supreme	..	„	84	„	295
Chop Suey	.. ..	„	77	„	270
Madras Curry	.. ..	„	76	„	269
Mexican Chilli	..	„	83	„	292
Mild Curry	.. ..	„	80	„	282
Paella Style	.. ..	„	88	„	309
Soya Mince with Onion	..	„	95	„	334
BIRD'S EYE *(frozen)*					
'Burgers'					
Original Beefburgers	..	each	150	—	—
Value Burgers	..	„	100	—	—

Meats, Savoury Pies

Food	Quantities	Calories	Quantities	Calories
100% Beefburgers ..	„	190	—	—
Quarter Pounders ..	„	300	—	—
Steakhouse Grill, beef ..	„	295	—	—
'MenuMaster'				
Beef Curry with Rice ..	1 packet	380	—	—
Beef Stew & Dumpling ..	„	240	—	—
Braised Kidneys in Gravy ..	„	200	—	—
Chicken Curry with Rice ..	„	400	—	—
Chicken & Mushroom Casserole ..	„	160	—	—
Chicken Supreme with Rice ..	„	460	—	—
Chilli Con Carne with Rice ..	„	375	—	—
Faggots in Rich Sauce	13 oz tray	690	—	—
Gravy & Lean Roast Beef	4 oz packet	95	—	—
Gravy & Roast Chicken ..	8 oz packet	190	—	—
Liver with Onion & Gravy	1 packet	190	—	—
Minced Beef with Veg. in Gravy ..	„	150	—	—
Paella, Seafood & Chicken	„	320	—	—
Prawn Curry with Rice ..	„	350	—	—
Roast Beef Dinner ..	„	360	—	—
Savoury Rissoles ..	each	170	—	—
'Pies, Flans & Pancakes'				
Beef Pie, Value ..	1 pie	370	—	—
Beefsteak & Veg. Pie ..	„	350	—	—
Cheese, Egg & Bacon Flan	5 oz	460	—	—
Cheese, Egg & Onion Flan	5 oz	460	—	—
Chicken Pie	1 pie	410	—	—
Chicken & Mushroom Pie	„	350	—	—
Minced Beef & Veg. Pie ..	„	410	—	—
Pancakes,				
Cheese & Ham ..	one	110	—	—
Chicken & Mushroom ..	„	110	—	—

Food			Quantities	Calories	Quantities	Calories
Minced Beef	..		one	100	—	—
Steak & Kidney Pie	..		1 pie	370	—	—
'Snacks'						
Brunchies	..	..	one	130	—	—
Cheesies	..	..	,,	60	—	—
Chicklets	..	..	,,	130	—	—
BRAINS						
Beefburgers with Onion	..		each	137	100 g	209
Beefsteak Pie	..	..	1/4 pie	308	,,	311
Cottage Pie	..		each	451	,,	134
Faggots in Rich Sauce	..		1 oz	44	,,	153
Family Chicken Pie	..		1/4 pie	240	,,	241
Family Shepherds Pie	..		each	609	100 g	122
Steak & Kidney Pie	..		1/4 pie	337	,,	338
CAMPBELLS						
'Meatball Products'						
In Curry Sauce	..		1 oz	34	100 g	119
In Gravy	..	..	,,	23	,,	80
In Onion Gravy	..		,,	25	,,	89
In Tomato Sauce	..		,,	27	,,	97
'Omelette Mates'						
Chicken & Mushroom	..		,,	19	,,	67
Mushroom	..	..	,,	11	,,	40
Tomato Bacon & Ham	..		,,	30	,,	106
'Stews'						
Beef Stew	..	..	,,	20	,,	70
Chicken Stew	..	..	,,	19	,,	66
Minced Beef & Vegetable	..		,,	28	,,	99
Steak & Kidney Stew	..		,,	18	,,	64

Meats, Savoury Pies

Food	Quantities	Calories	Quantities	Calories
CHAMBOURCY				
'Snack Meals'				
Chicken & Pineapple	1 oz	41	100 g	144
Curried Prawn	,,	40	,,	140
Salami	,,	72	,,	255
CHEF				
Baked Beans w/Hamburgers	—	—	100 g	122
Baked Beans w/Pork				
Sausages	—	—	,,	124
CROSSE AND BLACKWELL				
'Cook in the Pot'				
Beef Carbonade	1 oz	115	100 g	408
Beef Goulash	,,	108	,,	380
Beef Stroganoff	,,	119	,,	418
Chicken Chasseur	,,	110	,,	389
Chili-con-carne	,,	108	,,	382
Fish Bonne Femme	,,	108	,,	382
Lamb Ragout	,,	110	,,	389
'Meat Products'				
Ham & Beef Roll	,,	64	,,	226
Ham & Chicken Roll	,,	62	,,	220
Ham & Tongue Roll	,,	77	,,	270
'Ready Meals & Snacks'				
Beef Curry w/Sep. Rice	,,	35	,,	125
Chicken Curry w/Sep.				
Rice	,,	27	,,	96
Chili Con Carne	,,	35	,,	125
Faggots 'N' Peas	,,	32	,,	112
London Grill	,,	45	,,	157
Macaroni Cheese	,,	29	,,	102

Food	Quantities	Calories	Quantities	Calories
'Canned'				
Baked Beans in Tomato Sauce	—	—	100 g	96
FINDUS				
All Beef Quarterpounders ..	1 oz	80	100 g	283
90% Beefburgers ..	,,	80	,,	283
Beef Grillsteaks ..	,,	66	,,	233
Beef Pie, 1lb	,,	61	,,	216
Chicken Pie	,,	67	,,	236
Chicken & Veg. Pie, 1lb ..	,,	54	,,	190
Cornish Pasties ..	,,	79	,,	278
Crepes,				
Beef Burgundy ..	,,	40	,,	140
Chicken with Mushrooms ..	,,	38	,,	135
Curry,				
Beef (sauce only) ..	,,	27	,,	96
Chicken (sauce only) ..	,,	33	,,	115
Veg. & Prawn (sauce only) ..	,,	20	,,	69
Double Decker,				
Beef	,,	65	,,	230
Sausage	,,	55	,,	196
Flan,				
Egg, Cheese & Bacon ..	,,	68	,,	239
French Mushroom ..	,,	63	,,	224
French Onion ..	,,	66	,,	231
Moussaka	,,	30	,,	107
Pancakes,				
Cheddar Cheese ..	,,	54	,,	191
Chicken & Bacon ..	,,	40	,,	142
Chicken Curry ..	,,	45	,,	160

Meats, Savoury Pies

Food	Quantities	Calories	Quantities	Calories
Minced Beef	1 oz	45	100 g	160
Smoky Bacon .. ,,		40	,,	140
Roast Beef in Gravy .. ,,		23	,,	82
Sausages,				
Pork & Beef .. ,,		75	,,	263
Pork Chipolatas .. ,,		83	,,	293
Shepherds Pie .. .. ,,		34	,,	121
Steak & Kidney Pie .. ,,		64	,,	225
Toad in the Hole .. ,,		59	,,	207
FRAY BENTOS				
Chicken & Mushroom Pie	1 oz	56	100 g	196
Chicken & Mushroom Pie				
Filling .. .. .. ,,		30	,,	106
Corned Beef .. .. ,,		61	,,	215
Minced Steak & Onion Pie				
Filling .. ,,		56	,,	196
Savoury Minced Beef w/onions ,,		48	,,	168
Steak & Kidney Pie Filling .. ,,		42	,,	147
Steak & Kidney Pie .. ,,		62	,,	220
Steak & Kidney Pudding .. ,,		60	,,	212
Steak & Mushroom Pie				
Filling .. ,,		41	,,	144
Steak & Onion Pie Filling .. ,,		44	,,	156
Vegetable & Steak Pie .. ,,		52	,,	185
Vegetable & Steak Pie Filling .. ,,		33	,,	115
GOLDEN WONDER				
'Pot casserole'				
Beef	each	270	—	—
Chicken .. .. ,,		262	—	—
Lamb .. .. .. ,,		264	—	—

Food	Quantities	Calories	Quantities	Calories
GRANOSE				
Bologna	—	—	425 g	709
Dinner Balls	—	—	400 g	902
Fricassee	—	—	400 g	479
Frikaletts	—	—	425 g	505
Lentil & Veg. Casserole	—	—	425 g	384
Meatless Savoury Cutlets	—	—	42 g	374
Mexican Bean Stew	—	—	425 g	524
Nut Loaf	—	—	425 g	748
Nuttolene	—	—	284 g	284
Sausalatas	—	—	284 g	389
Savoury puddings	—	—	312 g	645
Soya Bean Pate	—	—	205 g	270
Tender Bits	—	—	425 g	335
Vegelinks	—	—	425 g	709
HEINZ				
Baked Beans w/Tomato Sauce	1 oz	20	100 g	72
Baked Beans w/Pork Sausages	,,	36	,,	126
Curried Beans w/Sultanas	,,	25	,,	87
'Take 5 Retort Pouch Meals'*				
Beef Curry w/Rice	,,	24	,,	83
Beef Goulash w/Rice	,,	22	,,	77
Chicken Curry w/Rice	,,	19	,,	66
INTERNATIONAL				
Baked Beans in Tomato Sauce	1 oz	28	100 g	100
Beefburgers (frozen)	,,	75	,,	265

* Footnote: These figures do not include nutritional content of rice.

Meats, Savoury Pies

Food		Quantities	Calories	Quantities	Calories
KRAFT					
Beef & Onion Slices	..	each	366	100 g	303
Beefburgers w/onion	..	,,	104	,,	209
Cheese & Onion Pies	..	,,	394	,,	277
Cheese & Ham Pies	..	,,	399	,,	281
Cheeseburgers	..	,,	173	,,	344
Chicken Pies	.. ..	,,	385	,,	340
Chicken & Mushroom Pies		,,	348	,,	272
Cornish Pasties	..	,,	302	,,	322
Cornish Pasties, traditional		,,	378	,,	333
Hamburgers w/onion	..	,,	104	,,	209
Meat & Vegetable Pies	..	,,	402	,,	354
Minced Beef & Onion Pies		,,	334	,,	261
Ploughmans Pasties	..	,,	433	,,	305
Sausage Rolls,					
Cheese Pastry	..	,,	107	,,	393
Cocktail	.. ..	,,	112	,,	393
King Size	.. ..	,,	220	,,	387
Steak & Kidney Pies	..	,,	442	,,	391
Steak & Kidney Puddings	..	,,	340	,,	282
MAPLETONS					
Nut Luncheon	..	—	—	142 g	542
Savormix	.. ..	—	—	100 g	425
MARKS AND SPENCERS *(canned)*					
Chicken in Jelly	..	1 oz	51	100 g	180
Chunky Chicken	..	,,	43	,,	150
Chunky Steak	.. ..	,,	50	,,	176
Cured Pork	.. ..	,,	77	,,	270
Cured Turkey	.. ..	,,	43	,,	150

Food	Quantities	Calories	Quantities	Calories
Curried Chicken	1 oz	34	100 g	120
Danish Ham	,,	34	,,	120
Minced Beef	,,	65	,,	229
(Delicatessen Dept.)				
Bavarian Ham Sausage	,,	45	,,	160
Bierwurst	,,	57	,,	200
Danish Ham	,,	37	,,	130
Honey Roast Ham	,,	49	,,	173
Parma Ham	,,	85	,,	300
Pork Shoulder	,,	35	,,	125
Roast Chicken	,,	61	,,	216
Roasted Ham	,,	62	,,	220
Roast Turkey	,,	55	,,	195
Salami	,,	139	,,	491
Smoked Mildcure Ham	,,	45	,,	160
Smoked Pork Loin	,,	57	,,	200
Smoked Spiced Ham	,,	62	,,	220
Smoked Sliced Gammon	,,	76	,,	269
Tandoori Chicken	,,	61	,,	216
(Pies)				
Beef & Mushroom Pasties	—	—	,,	262
Beef & Onion Pasties	—	—	,,	262
Beef Steak Pie w/Onion	—	—	,,	271
Beef Steak Pie, Topcrust	—	—	,,	203
Cheese, Bacon & Onion Flan	—	—	,,	298
Cheese & Onion Flan	—	—	,,	249
Cheese, Egg & Bacon Flan	—	—	,,	261
Chicken & Mushroom Pies	—	—	,,	282
Cornish Pasties, Pkt. of 4	—	—	,,	277
Cornish Pasties, singles	—	—	,,	231
Cornish Pasty, Traditional	—	—	,,	340

Meats, Savoury Pies

Food	Quantities	Calories	Quantities	Calories
Cottage Pies,				
Small	—	—	100 g	163
Large	—	—	,,	130
Family	—	—	,,	147
Minced Beef Pies,				
Small	—	—	,,	311
Large	—	—	,,	262
Top Crust	—	—	,,	282
Rich Pastry	—	—	,,	336
Roll	—	—	,,	324
Picnic Eggs	1 oz	94	,,	330
Pork & Egg Slice	,,	109	,,	385
Pork Pies	,,	123	,,	435
Pork Pies, crispbake	,,	108	,,	382
Sausage Rolls, Puff Pastry,				
Pork	,,	111	,,	390
Pork & Beef	,,	147	,,	519
Scotch Eggs	,,	85	,,	300
Scotch Pies	,,	71	,,	251
Steak & Kidney,				
Small	,,	86	,,	303
Rich Pastry	,,	87	,,	305
Turkey & Ham Pie, hot	,,	84	,,	295
Turkey in Rich Pastry, hot	,,	90	,,	318
(Poultry)				
Chicken,				
Battercrisp	,,	69	,,	242
Breast, Kiev	,,	91	,,	322
Breasts, Stuffed	,,	56	,,	197
Crumbed	,,	82	,,	289
Kebabs	,,	43	,,	153
Thighs	,,	60	,,	211

Food		Quantities	Calories	Quantities	Calories
Turkey,					
Boneless, Roast	..	1 oz	41	100 g	145
Breast w/Chestnut					
Stuffing	..	,,	66	,,	332
Breast Joint w/Pork Fat	..	,,	57	,,	201
Escalopes in					
Breadcrumbs	.. ..	,,	60	,,	212
Kebabs	.. ..	,,	25	,,	88
Loaf with Bacon	..	,,	46	,,	164
Medallions	.. ..	,,	58	,,	204
Sausages,					
Pork (average)	..	,,	123	,,	435
Pork & Beef	..	,,	95	,,	333
Skinless	.. ..	,,	96	,,	338
MATTESSONS					
Black Pudding	..	1 oz	102	100 g	359
Bratwurst	.. ..	,,	95	,,	334
Frankfurters	..	,,	101	,,	355
Chopped Pork & Ham	..	,,	94	,,	331
Garlic Sausage	..	,,	75	,,	264
German Sausage	..	,,	69	,,	243
Ham Sausage	..	,,	38	,,	134
Honey Roast Ham	..	,,	53	,,	186
Liver Sausage	..	,,	75	,,	264
Lunch Tongue	..	,,	74	,,	260
Maryland Ham	..	,,	32	,,	113
Old Smokey Ham	..	,,	67	,,	236
Polony	.. ..	,,	70	,,	246
Pork Luncheon Meat	..	,,	90	,,	317
Silverside	.. ..	,,	148	,,	169

Meats, Savoury Pies

Food	Quantities	Calories	Quantities	Calories
PREWETTS				
Beef Flavoured Chunks & Mince	1 oz	79	100 g	279
Brazilian Mix	,,	116	,,	407
Natural Flavoured Mince	,,	81	,,	287
Rissole Mixture	,,	116	,,	407
Smokey Snaps	,,	125	,,	441
PRINCES *(canned)*				
Chopped Ham & Pork	1 oz	95	100 g	333
Corned Beef	,,	66	,,	232
Ham	,,	42	,,	147
Pork Luncheon Meat	,,	112	,,	395
PROTOVEG MENU				
Farmhouse Soya Stew	4 oz	404	—	—
Mixed Soya & Onion	5 oz	507	—	—
Soya Bolognese Mix	4 oz	388	—	—
ROSS *(frozen)*				
American Hamburgers	1 oz	91	100 g	320
Beefburgers	,,	77	,,	270
Beefburgers 100%	,,	91	,,	320
Beef Grills	,,	94	,,	330
Breast of Chicken Roll	,,	43	,,	150
Breast of Turkey	,,	40	,,	140
Chicken Portion	,,	62	,,	220
Chicken Portions (cooked)	,,	68	,,	240
Chopped Veal Steaks	,,	68	,,	240
Cornish Pasties	,,	80	,,	280
Faggots in Rich Sauce	,,	51	,,	180

Food	Quantities	Calories	Quantities	Calories
Family Meals,				
Shepherds Pie	1 oz	28	100 g	100
Steak & Kidney Pie	,,	57	,,	200
Family Pies,				
Beef	,,	27	,,	270
Chicken	,,	74	,,	260
Meat & Potato	,,	80	,,	280
Fried Chicken Drumsticks	,,	60	,,	210
Gravy with Sliced Roast				
Beef	,,	28	,,	100
Grillsteaks	,,	91	,,	320
Hamburgers with Onions	,,	74	,,	260
Jumboburgers	,,	68	,,	240
Meatballs	,,	68	,,	240
Pizza, average all flavours	,,	65	,,	230
Sausages, average all flavours	,,	82	,,	290
Sausage Rolls	,,	88	,,	310
Scotch Fritters with Beans/				
Cheese	,,	70	,,	245
Shepherds Pie	,,	34	,,	120
Southern Fried Chicken				
Portions	,,	68	,,	240
Cumberland Pie	1 meal	280	—	—
Hamburgers	,,	310	—	—
Irish Stew	,,	290	—	—
Lamb Casserole	,,	260	—	—
Liver Slices	,,	290	—	—
Meat Balls in Gravy	,,	330	—	—
Minced Beef	,,	300	—	—
Minced Beef & Vegetable				
Pie	,,	400	—	—
Pork & Apple Casserole	,,	220	—	—

Meats, Savoury Pies

Food	Quantities	Calories	Quantities	Calories
Sausages	1 meal	390	—	—
Sliced Beef	,,	230	—	—
Sliced Lamb	,,	260	—	—
Sliced Pork	,,	250	—	—
Steak & Kidney Pie	,,	370	—	—
Stewed Steak	,,	250	—	—
Sliced Turkey	,,	240	—	—
Individual Meals				
Beef Casserole	,,	260	—	—
Beef Hot Pot	,,	270	—	—
Boiled Beef & Carrots	,,	250	—	—
Chicken Casserole	,,	180	—	—
Chicken Curry	,,	220	—	—
Chicken Pie	,,	300	—	—
Chicken & Stuffing	,,	230	—	—
Cottage Pie	,,	280	—	—
SAFEWAY *(fresh)*				
Beef Loaf	1 oz	82	100 g	290
Black Pudding	,,	88	,,	311
Breaded Beef Grill	,,	82	,,	290
Breaded Pork Grill	,,	102	,,	360
Bridie	,,	82	,,	290
Faggots	,,	47	,,	166
Fruit Pudding	,,	108	,,	381
Haggis	,,	92	,,	324
Lorne Sausage	,,	93	,,	326
Mini Scotch Pie	,,	58	,,	203
Ranch Burgers	,,	89	,,	315
Scotch Minced Beef Pie	,,	71	,,	252
Scotch Pie	,,	60	,,	213
White Pudding	,,	134	,,	472

Food	Quantities	Calories	Quantities	Calories
(frozen)				
Beefburgers	1 oz	85	100 g	298
Beef Croquettes	,,	71	,,	250
SOYAPRO PROTEIN FOODS				
Beef-like Flavour	1 oz	59	100 g	207
Chicken-like Flavour	,,	69	,,	242
Soya Wieners	,,	63	,,	221
SPAR				
Baked Beans	1 oz	24	100 g	85
TESCO *(canned)*				
Baked Beans	1 oz	30	100 g	105
Baked Beans & Sausages	,,	35	,,	123
Beefburgers in Gravy	,,	41	,,	145
Chicken Curry	,,	44	,,	155
Chicken Pie	,,	60	,,	212
Chicken in White Sauce	,,	71	,,	250
Chopped Ham & Pork	,,	96	,,	339
Hamburgers in Gravy	,,	41	,,	145
Hot Dogs (mini)	,,	60	,,	210
Hot Dog Sausages	,,	52	,,	182
Irish Stew	,,	35	,,	124
Meatballs w/Onion	,,	34	,,	120
Meatballs in Tom Sauce	,,	29	,,	101
Minced Beef & Onion	,,	46	,,	163
Minced Beef Pie	,,	103	,,	364
Minced Beef Pie Filling	,,	35	,,	124
Pork Kidneys, Braised	,,	28	,,	100

Meats, Savoury Pies

Food		Quantities	Calories	Quantities	Calories
Pork Luncheon Meat	..	1 oz	91	100 g	321
Pork Sausages in Lard	..	,,	89	,,	312
Steak & Kidney Pie,					
Large	.. ..	,,	56	,,	198
Small	.. ..	,,	50	,,	177
Stewed Steak in Gravy	..	,,	47	,,	167
(Frozen)					
Beefburgers	..	,,	45	,,	157
Beef & Vegetable Pie	..	,,	79	,,	280
Chicken Pie	.. ..	,,	81	,,	286
Shepherds Pie	..	,,	31	,,	110
Steak & Kidney Pie	..	,,	81	,,	286
(Pies)					
Beef & Kidney Pie	..	,,	82	,,	288
Beef & Kidney Pudding,					
Large	.. ..	,,	78	,,	274
Small	.. ..	,,	83	,,	294
Beef & Onion Pies, all sizes		,,	79	,,	277
Cheese & Onion Flan	..	,,	87	,,	307
Chicken & Vegetable Pie	..	,,	67	,,	236
Cornish Pasty	.. ..	,,	80	,,	281
Cottage Pie	.. ..	,,	56	,,	198
Meat & Potato Pie	..	,,	77	,,	273
Sausage Rolls	.. ..	,,	117	,,	412
Sausages,					
Pork	.. .. ..	,,	97	,,	342
Pork & Herb	..	,,	107	,,	376
Premium	.. ..	,,	94	,,	331
Skinless	.. ..	,,	97	,,	342
Smoked	.. ..	,,	102	,,	358
Sausage Meat	.. ..	,,	98	,,	345
Sausage Meat & Herbs	..	,,	105	,,	371

Food	Quantities	Calories	Quantities	Calories
WAITROSE *(canned)*				
Baked Beans	1 oz	26	100 g	91
Chopped Pork & Ham ..	,,	46	,,	162
Hamburgers	,,	46	,,	162
Stewed Steak	,,	40	,,	141
(fresh)				
Chopped Pork & Ham ..	,,	97	,,	341
Pork Luncheon Meat ..	,,	95	,,	334
Sausages,				
Beef	,,	82	,,	289
Pork	,,	97	,,	341
(frozen)				
Beefburgers	,,	50	,,	176
Steak & Kidney Pie ..	,,	86	,,	303

Pasta, Pizza and Rice

This is a new section for this edition as there are now so many canned and packet products available. Not the healthiest or lowest in calories it is still permissible to have things from this section in moderation.

Food	Quantities	Calories	Quantities	Calories
BIRD'S EYE *(frozen)*				
French Bread Pizza ..	one	330	—	—
French Bread Pizza, de luxe	,,	360	—	—
Lasagne	9 oz	315	—	
Pizza,				
Ham & Mushroom (265 g)	one	640	—	—
Tomato & Cheese (93 g)	,,	270	—	—
Spaghetti Bolognese ..	1 packet	370	—	—
BUITONI				
Dry Pasta (all shapes) ..	1 oz	·95	100 g	334
Canned,				
Canelloni	1 can	388	—	—
Ravioli	,,	292	—	—
CROSSE AND BLACKWELL				
'Alutray Meals'				
Canelloni	—	—	100 g	103
Lasagne	—	—	,,	112

Food	Quantities	Calories	Quantities	Calories
Tortellini	—	—	,,	106
2-minute Noodles, Beef & Chicken ..	1 oz	30	,,	106
canned)				
Spaghetti Rings & Alphabetti ..	—	—	,,	61
Straight Spaghetti ..	—	—	,,	57
Pasta Choice'				
Average, all flavours ..	1 oz	99	,,	348
INDUS				
Cannelloni	1 oz	27	100 g	96
Lasagne	,,	28	,,	100
French Bread Pizzas'				
Bacon Peppers & Mushrooms ..	,,	55	,,	192
Italian Style Sausage ..	,,	52	,,	183
Savoury Barbecue Beef ..	,,	63	,,	223
Tomato & Cheese ..	,,	65	,,	228
Crusty Bun Pizza' ..	,,	66	,,	231
Crispy Base Pizza'				
Cheese & Tomato ..	,,	59	,,	208
Ham	,,	47	,,	168
GOLDEN WONDER				
Pot Noodles' (including sauce) ..				
Beef & Tomato ..	1 pot	386	—	—
Cheese & Tomato ..	,,	353	—	—
Chicken & Mushroom ..	,,	388	—	—
Curry Flavour	,,	393	—	—
Sweet & Sour	,,	355	—	—

Pasta and Rice

Food	Quantities	Calories	Quantities	Calories
HEINZ				
Macaroni Cheese	—	—	100 g	123
Noodle Doodles	—	—	,,	63
Ravioli in Beef & Tomato Sauce	—	—	,,	90
Ravioli in Tomato Sauce	—	—	,,	96
Spaghetti Bolognese	—	—	,,	88
Spaghetti & Hoops in Tomato Sauce	—	—	,,	67
Spaghetti Shells in Spicy Sauce	—	—	,,	77
INTERNATIONAL				
Spaghetti & Rings in Tomato Sauce	—	—	100 g	59
KRAFT				
Cheesey Pasta (as prepared)	1 oz	48	100 g	169
MARKS AND SPENCER *(frozen)*				
Minced Beef Lasagne	—	—	100 g	95
Pizzas, Small				
Marguerita	1 oz	62	,,	218
Tomato, Cheese & Onion	,,	56	,,	203
Pizzas, Large				
Bacon, Mushroom & Peppers	,,	52	,,	182
Cheeese & Tomato	,,	68	,,	239

Food	Quantities	Calories	Quantities	Calories
PREWETT				
'Heat & Serve Main Meals'				
Cannelloni	—	—	100 g	82
Ravioli	—	—	,,	62
Tortellini	—	—	,,	68
RECORD				
Wholewheat Pasta (all shapes)	—	—	100 g	327
SAFEWAY (*Pizzas*)				
Cheese & Onion	1 oz	66	100 g	233
Cheese & Tomato	,,	70	,,	247
Cheese & Tomato French Bread	,,	59	,,	207
Ham & Mushroom	,,	64	,,	227
TESCO (*canned*)				
Ravioli	—	—	100 g	70
Spaghetti Lengths & Letters	—	—	,,	80
Spaghetti Hoops	—	—	,,	66
Rice				
BATCHELOR				
'Savoury Rice'				
Beef	1 packet	406	—	—
Chicken	,,	435	—	—
Golden	,,	438	—	—
Mild Curry	,,	451	—	—
Mixed Vegetables	,,	446	—	—
Sweet & Sour	,,	501	—	—
Tropical Fruit	,,	432	—	—

Pasta and Rice

Food	Quantities	Calories	Quantities	Calories
CROSSE AND BLACKWELL				
'Alutray Meals', Paella	—	—	100 g	175
'Rice Things' (reconstituted)				
Average, all flavours	—	—	,,	106
GOLDEN WONDER				
'Pot Rice'				
Chicken Curry	1 pot	264	—	—
Savoury Beef	,,	254	—	—
Spicy Tomato	,,	251	—	—
KELLOGG				
'Boil in Bag' Rice	1 oz	93	100 g	328
SAFEWAY (*Rice*)				
Curry Savoury Rice	1 oz	98	100 g	346
Spanish Savoury Rice	,,	96	,,	340
Tomato Savoury Rice	,,	95	,,	334
TESCO				
'Savoury Rice'				
Beef	—	—	100 g	345
Chicken	—	—	,,	350
All other flavours, average	—	—	,,	330

Salads

Another new section for this edition! Although containing more calories than fresh produce, these ready-to-eat salads make a very satisfying 'diet' lunch accompanied by cold meats, cottage cheese or, perhaps, a hard-boiled egg.

Food	Quantities	Calories	Quantities	Calories
CHAMBOURCY				
Coleslaw	—	—	100 g	150
EDENVALE				
Chicken & Sweetcorn	1 oz	44	100 g	156
Coarse Cut Coleslaw	,,	35	,,	125
Coleslaw	,,	36	,,	126
Country Salad	,,	35	,,	125
Potato	,,	41	,,	146
Prawn	,,	43	,,	153
Spanish	,,	31	,,	110
Spicy	,,	40	,,	141
Tropical	,,	37	,,	130
Vegetable	,,	40	,,	141
Vinaigrette	,,	9	,,	33
HEINZ *(canned)*				
Coleslaw	—	—	100 g	127
Potato Salad	—	—	,,	191
Vegetable Salad	—	—	,,	145

Salads

Food		Quantities	Calories	Quantities	Calories
MARKS AND SPENCER					
Beetroot in Vinaigrette	..	1 oz	47	100 g	165
Florida	.. .. ..	,,	58	,,	205
Pasta	.. .. ..	,,	82	,,	290
Potato	.. .. ..	,,	91	,,	322
Vegetable	.. .. ..	,,	75	,,	265
Waldorf	.. ..	,,	85	,,	298
MATTESONS					
Celery, Apple & Orange	..	1 oz	55	100 g	194
Coleslaw	.. ..	,,	48	,,	169
Coleslaw in Vinaigrette	..	,,	23	,,	81
Crispy Celery & Cucumber		,,	23	,,	81
French Salad	.. ..	,,	23	,,	81
Ham Salad	.. ..	,,	60	,,	211
Potato Salad	.. ..	,,	48	,,	169
Prawn Cocktail	..	,,	55	,,	194
Snack Salad	.. ..	,,	40	,,	141
Spanish Salad	.. ..	,,	32	,,	113
Spring Salad	.. ..	,,	50	,,	176
Vegetable Salad	..	,,	34	,,	120
ST. IVEL					
Coleslaw	.. ..	1 oz	34	100 g	120
Coleslaw in Vinaigrette	..	,,	27	,,	95
Crispy Vegetable in Vinaigrette		,,	20	,,	70
Florida	.. .. ..	,,	28	,,	100
Prawn	.. .. ..	,,	44	,,	155
Waldorf	.. ..	,,	38	,,	135

Food		Quantities	Calories	Quantities	Calories
TESCO *(canned)*					
Beetroot	.. ..	1 oz	39	100 g	137
Coleslaw (low cal.)	..	,,	15	,,	53
Potato	.. .. ..	,,	44	,,	155
Vegetable	.. ..	,,	43	,,	152
(fresh)					
Coleslaw,					
Plain	.. .. ..	,,	36	,,	126
Low cal.	.. .. ..	,,	14	,,	48
Vinaigrette	.. ..	,,	17	,,	60
Mixed in French Dressing	..	,,	21	,,	73
Florida	.. .. ..	,,	36	,,	126
Potato	.. .. ..	,,	41	,,	145

Sauces, Salad Dressings, Pickles and Relishes

Used sparingly, sauces do add variety to plain foods essential to *measure them carefully* as the calories add up all too quickly. Pickles, on the other hand, are very low in calorific content (except sweet pickles), and are useful to munch on when on a strict diet.

Food		Quantities	Calories	Quantities	Calories
BAXTER					
'Cooking-in-Sauces'					
Burgundy Wine Sauce	..	1 oz	59	100 g	209
Madeira Wine Sauce	..	,,	70	,,	245
Madras Hot Curry Sauce	..	,,	87	,,	307
Medium Curry Sauce	..	,,	87	,,	307
Sauce Provencale	..	,,	113	,,	398
Sweet & Sour Sauce	..	,,	107	,,	377
White Wine Sauce	..	,,	111	,,	390
BAXTERS					
Beetroot, Pickled (average)		1 oz	10	100 g	35
Beetroot & Redcurrant					
Relish	..	,,	48	,,	169
Country Pickle	..	,,	47	,,	165
Cranberry Sauce, Jellied	..	,,	71	,,	251

Food	Quantities	Calories	Quantities	Calories
Cranberry Sauce, Whole Fruit	1 oz	39	100 g	139
Mild Mustard Pickle	,,	41	,,	143
Mixed Fruit Pickle	,,	49	,,	173
Mint Jelly	,,	73	,,	259
Mint Sauce, concentrated & ready	,,	43	,,	150
Tomato Pickle	,,	53	,,	188
BIRDS				
Gravy Mix	1 oz	6	100 g	21
BONNE CUISINE				
Sauce au Poivre	1 oz	109	100 g	383
Sauce Chasseur	,,	98	,,	345
Sauce Basquaise	,,	104	,,	360
Sauce Hollandaise	,,	109	,,	384
Sauce Madeira	,,	102	,,	359
Sauce Paysan	,,	99	,,	348
BRANSTON				
Fruity Sauce	1 oz	26	100 g	90
Pickle, Sweet	,,	37	,,	131
Spicy Sauce	,,	32	,,	112
Tomato Chutney	,,	41	,,	144
BUITONI				
Bolognese Sauce	1 can	144	—	—
Milanese Sauce	,,	142	—	—
Napolitan Sauce	,,	76	—	—
Tomato Puree	1 tube	94	—	—

Sauces, Salad Dressings, Pickles

Food	Quantities	Calories	Quantities	Calories
CAMPBELLS 'Spaghetti Sauces'				
Bolognese	1 oz	25	100 g	90
Tomato	,,	21	,,	76
Tomato & Mushroom	,,	19	,,	68
'Prego Sauces'				
Bolognese	,,	28	,,	100
Napolitan	,,	26	,,	93
Pizza	,,	21	,,	76
CHEF				
Tomato Ketchup	1 oz	31	100 g	109
COLMANS				
Apple Sauce	1 oz	23	100 g	80
'Casserole Mixes'				
Beef Bourguignon	,,	99	,,	350
Beef Provencale	,,	79	,,	280
Beef Strogonoff	,,	91	,,	320
Chicken Chasseur	,,	70	,,	245
Chilli con Carne	,,	84	,,	295
Coq au Vin	,,	70	,,	245
Goulash	,,	78	,,	275
Navarin of Lamb	,,	92	,,	325
Pork Piquant	,,	84	,,	295
Cranberry Sauce & Wine	,,	61	,,	215
Creamed Horseradish	,,	60	,,	210
'Curry Mixes'				
Korma, Madras & Vindaloo	,,	95	,,	335
Tandoori Marinade	,,	61	,,	215
'Dry Sauce Mixes'				
Apple	,,	108	,,	380

Food			Quantities	Calories	Quantities	Calories
Barbecue	..	.. ..	1 oz	88	100 g	310
Beef Seasoning		..	,,	89	,,	315
Bread	..	.. ..	,,	91	,,	320
Cheese	..	.. ..	,,	118	,,	415
Chicken Seasoning		..	,,	102	,,	360
Curry	..	.. ..	,,	99	,,	350
Mushroom		.. ..	,,	95	,,	335
Onion	..	.. ..	,,	67	,,	235
Parsley	..	.. ..	,,	102	,,	360
Spaghetti		.. ..	,,	105	,,	370
Sweet & Sour		.. ..	,,	91	,,	320
White	..	.. ..	,,	108	,,	380
Fresh Garden Mint		..	,,	7	,,	25
Gravy Pot (concentrate)		..	,,	152	,,	535
Horseradish Relish		..	,,	28	,,	100
'Master Sauces'						
Bearnaise		.. ..	,,	104	,,	365
Borderline		.. ..	,,	95	,,	335
Mornay		.. ..	,,	105	,,	370
Provencale	..	.. ..	,,	92	,,	325
Mint Jelly		.. ..	,,	96	,,	340
Prawn Cocktail Sauce		..	,,	111	,,	390
Redcurrant Sauce		..	,,	82	,,	290
Sauce Tartare		.. ..	,,	72	,,	255
CROSSE AND BLACKWELL						
Sauces'						
Bolognese		.. ..	1 oz	20	100 g	70
Cheese	..	.. ..	,,	30	,,	106
Curry	..	.. ..	,,	27	,,	95
Sweet & Sour		.. ..	,,	32	,,	112
Salad Cream		.. ..	,,	98	,,	346

Sauces, Salad Dressings, Pickles

Food		Quantities	Calories	Quantities	Calories
EPICURE *(Pickles)*					
Beetroot, baby sliced	..	1 oz	8	100 g	29
Beetroot, sweet sliced	..	,,	13	,,	46
Gherkins	.. ..	,,	5	,,	17
Mixed	.. .. ..	—	—	,,	4
Mustard Piccalilli	..	1 oz	6	,,	23
Onions	.. .. ..	,,	4	,,	14
Onions, sweet	.. ..	,,	7	,,	25
Red Cabbage	.. ..	,,	3	,,	12
Silverskin Onions	..	,,	4	,,	15
Sweet	.. .. ..	,,	38	,,	134
Sweet Piccalilli	..	,,	22	,,	77
Walnuts	.. ..	,,	20	,,	69
FLORA					
Sunflower Dressing	..1 Tablespoon	75	—	—	
HAPPY FARM					
Piccalilli	.. ..	1 oz	9	100 g	33
Sweet Pickle	.. ..	,,	38	,,	134
Tomato & Apple Chutney	..	,,	48	,,	170
HAYWARD *(Pickles)*					
Beetroot	.. ..	1 oz	8	100 g	40
Gherkins	.. ..	,,	1	,,	5
Mixed Pickle	.. ..	,,	3	,,	9
Piccalilli	.. ..	,,	8	,,	29
Pickled Onions	..	,,	4	,,	16
Red Cabbage	.. ..	,,	3	,,	10
Silverskin Onions	..	,,	6	,,	20
Sweet Military Pickle	..	,,	37	,,	130
Sweet Piccalilli	..	,,	21	,,	75
Walnuts	.. ..	,,	23	,,	80

Food		Quantities	Calories	Quantities	Calories
HEINZ					
French Dressing	..	1 oz	147	100 g	519
Ideal Sauce	.. ..	,,	33	,,	115
Mayonaise	.. ..	,,	145	,,	512
Mild Mustard Pickle	..	,,	37	,,	130
Piccalilli	.. ..	,,	21	,,	73
Ploughman's Pickle	..	,,	39	,,	136
Salad Cream	.. ..	,,	89	,,	312
Tomato Ketchup	..	,,	31	,,	108
Tomato Pickle	..	,,	32	,,	112
Yoghurt Dressing	..	,,	81	,,	285
HELLMAN'S					
Blue Cheese Dressing	..	1 oz	214	100 g	755
Curry Dressing	..	,,	172	,,	606
Mayonnaise, all flavours	..	,,	204	,,	720
Soured Cream & Chives Dressing	.. ..	,,	161	,,	567
Thousand Island	.. ..	,,	155	,,	548
Yoghurt & Cucumber	..	,,	163	,,	575
HP					
Al Sauce	.. ..	1 oz	35	100 g	124
'Country Cooking Sauces'					
Brown Ale	.. ..	,,	13	,,	45
Cider	.. .. ..	,,	13	,,	47
Curry	.. .. ..	,,	14	,,	49
Red Wine	.. ..	,,	12	,,	43
Tomato & Herb	..	,,	9	,,	31
Curry Concentrate	..	,,	45	,,	160
Daddies Favourite sauce	..	,,	17	,,	60
Daddies Tomato Ketchup	..	,,	30	,,	105

Sauces, Salad Dressings, Pickles

Food	Quantities	Calories	Quantities	Calories
Daddies Tomato Sauce ..	1 oz	19	100 g	66
Fruit Sauce	,,	34	,,	120
Fruity Sauce	,,	25	,,	90
HP Sauce	,,	21	,,	75
Mint Sauce	,,	24	,,	85
Private Label Salad Cream	,,	91	,,	320
Tomato Ketchup ..	,,	28	,,	100

INTERNATIONAL
'Pickles'

Food	Quantities	Calories	Quantities	Calories
Beetroot, Baby ..	1 oz	13	100 g	46
Beetroot, Sliced ..	,,	8	,,	29
Piccalilli	,,	6	,,	23
Pickled Onions ..	,,	4	,,	14
Red Cabbage	,,	3	,,	12
Sweet Pickle	,,	28	,,	154

'Sauces'

Food	Quantities	Calories	Quantities	Calories
Brown	,,	30	,,	105
Creamed Horseradish ..	,,	47	,,	165
Horseradish	,,	30	,,	106
Mayonnaise	,,	216	,,	760
Mint	,,	11	,,	38
Salad Cream	,,	111	,,	392
Seafood Dressing	,,	132	,,	466
Spaghetti	,,	106	,,	370
Tartare	,,	89	,,	314
Tomato Ketchup	,,	28	,,	100

'Stuffings'

Food	Quantities	Calories	Quantities	Calories
Parsley & Thyme	,,	101	,,	355
Sage & Onion	,,	97	,,	342

Food	Quantities	Calories	Quantities	Calories
KNORR				
Sauce Mixes'				
Apple	1 packet	98	—	—
Bread	,,	144	—	—
Cheese	,,	134	—	—
Korma Curry	,,	174	—	—
Onion	,,	96	—	—
Parsley	,,	70	—	—
Savoury White	,,	72	—	—
Seafood	,,	174	—	—
Spaghetti	,,	152	—	—
Stock Cubes'				
Gravy	1 cube	41	—	—
Other flavours, average	,,	33	—	—
Stuffing Mixes'				
Cider Apple & Herbs	1 oz	114	1 packet	360
Garlic & Herbs	,,	116	,,	369
Hazelnut & Herbs	,,	121	,,	383
Sage & Onion	,,	112	,,	356
KRAFT				
Salad Dressings'				
Chunky Blue Cheese	1 oz	127	100 g	446
Classic French	,,	145	,,	510
Coleslaw	,,	131	,,	461
Creamy Cucumber	,,	144	,,	508
Italian Garlic	,,	125	,,	439
Thousand Island	,,	118	,,	391
LEA AND PERRINS				
Worcestershire Sauce	1 oz	20	100 g	72

Sauces, Salad Dressings, Pickles

Food	Quantities	Calories	Quantities	Calories
LIBBY				
Tomato Ketchup ..	1 oz	30	100 g	106
MARKS AND SPENCER				
Beetroot Pickle ..	1 oz	12	100 g	44
Blue Cheese/Garlic Dressings ..	,,	187	,,	660
Irish Dressing, Red & White ..	,,	115	,,	405
Mayonaise	,,	204	,,	718
Onion Dressing w/Chives ..	,,	106	,,	372
Sunflower Oil Dressing ..	,,	255	,,	899
Thousand Island ..	,,	168	,,	590
Walnut Dressing ..	,,	118	,,	417
O.K.				
Fruity Sauce ..	1 oz	25	100 g	90
Mint Sauce ..	,,	14	,,	50
Spicy Sauce ..	,,	27	,,	95
Sunny Sauce ..	,,	24	,,	85
PAN-YAN				
Bramley Apple Sauce ..	1 oz	16	100 g	55
Garden Mint Sauce ..	,,	9	,,	32
Original Pickle ..	,,	45	,,	159
RAYNER/BURGESS				
Brown Sauce	1 oz	21	100 g	74
Cranberry Sauce ..	,,	38	,,	136
Creamed Horseradish ..	,,	53	,,	188
Hot Horseradish ..	,,	58	,,	203
Mango Chutney ..	,,	58	,,	203
Mayonnaise	,,	168	,,	592

Food	Quantities	Calories	Quantities	Calories
Mint Sauce	1 oz	17	100 g	59
Mushroom Ketchup ..	,,	3	,,	10
Prawn Cocktail ..	,,	85	,,	300
Relishes, average all flavours ..	,,	31	,,	108
Salad Dressing, Low Calorie ..	,,	33	,,	117
Sauce Tartare	,,	77	,,	270
Tomato Ketchup ..	,,	40	,,	140
SAFEWAY				
Horseradish	1 oz	16	100 g	55
Horseradish, creamed ..	,,	43	,,	150
Mayonaise	,,	218	,,	766
Pickle, clear mixed ..	,,	2	,,	8
Pickled Sliced Cucumber ..	,,	8	,,	28
Sauces'				
Fruity	,,	22	,,	79
Mint	,,	5	,,	17
Tartare	,,	78	,,	275
Sauce Mixes'				
Apple	,,	104	,,	365
Bread	,,	100	,,	352
Cheese	,,	119	,,	418
Onion	,,	103	,,	364
Parsley	,,	101	,,	356
White	,,	104	,,	366
TESCO				
Bolognese	1 oz	28	100 g	100
Chop	,,	23	,,	81
Fruit	,,	19	,,	67

Sauces, Salad Dressings, Pickles

Food			Quantities	Calories	Quantities	Calories
Horseradish, cream		..	1 oz	53	100 g	187
Horseradish, sauce		..	,,	35	,,	125
Mayonnaise	..	..	,,	216	,,	760
Mint Jelly	..	..	,,	75	,,	266
Mint Sauce	..	..	,,	28	,,	100
Prawn Cocktail		..	,,	91	,,	320
Salad Cream	..	..	,,	114	,,	402
Tartare ..	..	..	,,	79	,,	277
Tomato Ketchup		..	,,	25	,,	100
Vinegar & Oil	..	..	,,	43	,,	152

Savoury Spreads

In the previous edition these were listed in the 'jam' section. There are now enough available to warrant a section of their own. Also these should probably be substituted for a main meal and make another useful choice for a working lunch. But remember—not too much bread or crispbread with them!

Food	Quantities	Calories	Quantities	Calories
HEINZ				
Cucumber Spread ..	1 oz	62	100 g	219
Sandwich Spread ..	,,	68	,,	240
Toast Toppers'				
Chicken & Mushroom ..	,,	22	,,	79
Ham & Cheese ..	,,	55	,,	195
Mushroom & Bacon ..	,,	35	,,	123
Pizza	,,	20	,,	70
Turkey & Ham ..	,,	31	,,	109
INTERNATIONAL				
Pastes'				
Chicken & Meat Flavours ..	1 oz	66	100 g	232
Fish Flavours	,,	41	,,	144
MARKS AND SPENCER				
Beef, Country, Farmhouse, Ham ..	1 oz	85	100 g	300
Smoked Mackerel ..	,,	90	,,	318

Savoury Spreads

Food		Quantities	Calories	Quantities	Calories
MATTESONS					
Ardennes Pate	..	1 oz	110	100 g	387
Brussels Pate	.. ..	,,	117	,,	412
Crab Spreading Pate	..	,,	82	,,	289
Garlic Spreading Pate	..	,,	90	,,	317
Salmon Spreaing Pate	..	,,	82	,,	289
Kipper Spreading Pate	..	,,	72	,,	253
Turkey Pate	.. ..	,,	95	,,	334
PRINCES					
'Pates'					
Chicken Liver	.. ..	1 jar/can	310	—	—
Pork Liver	.. ..	,,	301	—	—
Smoked Ham	.. ..	,,	310	—	—
Turkey	.. .. ..	,,	315	—	—
'Pastes'					
Beef	.. .. ..	,,	161	—	—
Beef & Bacon	.. ..	,,	182	—	—
Chicken & Ham	..	,,	172	—	—
Crab	.. ..	,,	76	—	—
Salmon & Cucumber	..	,,	79	—	—
'Spreads'					
Beef	.. .. ..	,,	108	—	—
Crab	.. .. ..	,,	64	—	—
Fried Chicken	.. ..	,,	127	—	—
Ham	.. .. ..	,,	124	—	—
Lobster	.. ..	,,	63	—	—
Salmon	.. ..	,,	62	—	—
Smokey Bacon	..	,,	120	—	—

Soups

Soups make a very satisfying meal—particularly during cold weather—and, if care is exercised in choosing those with fewer calories, they are not fattening. The danger lies in adding either milk or butter, or eating hunks of French bread with the soup. But stick to a bowl of soup and a slice of bread with low-calorie spread and you will continue to lose weight.

Food	Quantities	Calories	Quantities	Calories
BATCHELORS				
'5 Minute Soups'				
Asparagus	1 oz	64	100 g	224
Barbecue Beef & Tomato	,,	48	,,	171
Chicken & Mushroom	,,	62	,,	219
Choice Celery	,,	53	,,	188
Country Chicken & Leek	,,	51	,,	181
Country Chicken Noodle	,,	44	,,	154
Farmers Thick Chicken	,,	66	,,	233
French Onion	,,	28	,,	99
Golden Lentil	,,	59	,,	207
Golden Vegetable	,,	62	,,	217
Harvest Vegetable & Chicken	,,	62	,,	217
Italian Tomato & Vegetable	,,	42	,,	148

Soups

Food	Quantities	Calories	Quantities	Calories
Minestrone	1 oz	43	100 g	153
Oxtail	,,	45	,,	159
Rich Cottage Vegetable ..	,,	55	,,	193
Rich Country Mushroom ..	,,	60	,,	211
Savoury Beef & Onion ..	,,	44	,,	154
Scotch Broth	,,	39	,,	137
Spring Vegetable ..	,,	25	,,	88
Thick Devon Onion ..	,,	50	,,	175
Thick Farmhouse Vegetable	,,	41	,,	146
Thick Lincoln Pea ..	,,	68	,,	241
Thick Savoury Vegetable ..	,,	56	,,	197
Traditional Tomato ..	,,	76	,,	267
Traditional Vegetable & Beef ..	,,	46	,,	164
'Cup-A-Soup'				
Asparagus	,,	28	,,	99
Beef & Tomato ..	,,	16	,,	58
Celery	,,	29	,,	104
Chicken	,,	29	,,	104
Chicken & Leek ..	,,	26	,,	91
Golden Vegetable ..	,,	20	,,	72
Mushroom	,,	33	,,	115
Onion	,,	32	,,	112
Oxtail	,,	22	,,	77
Tomato	,,	23	,,	83
Vegetable & Beef ..	,,	24	,,	85
'Cup-A-Soup' (Special)				
Barbecue Bacon & Tomato ..	,,	31	,,	108
Chicken & Vegetable ..	,,	32	,,	113
French Onion, Cheese & Croutons ..	,,	16	,,	58

Food		Quantities	Calories	Quantities	Calories
Minestrone w/Croutons	..	1 oz	20	100 g	70
Thick Mushroom	..	,,	31	,,	108
Tomato & Vegetable w/Croutons	..	.. ,,	31	,,	110
BAXTERS *(canned)*					
Beef Broth	.. ..	1 can	188	100 g	44
Chicken Broth	..	,,	141	,,	33
Cock-a-Leekie	..	,,	60	,,	14
Cream of Asparagus	..	,,	264	,,	62
Cream of Chicken	..	,,	241	,,	57
Cream of Game	..	,,	296	,,	70
Cream of Leek	..	,,	217	,,	51
Cream of Mushroom	..	,,	264	,,	62
Cream of Pheasant	..	,,	235	,,	55
Cream of Scampi	..	,,	275	,,	65
Cream of Tomato	..	,,	319	,,	74
Cream of Smoked Trout	..	,,	277	,,	65
Cream of Sweetcorn	..	,,	238	,,	56
Cream of Vegetable	..	,,	221	,,	52
Curried Beef	.. ..	,,	153	,,	36
French Onion	.. ..	,,	59	,,	14
Game Consomme	..	,,	49	,,	12
Highlander's Broth	..	,,	147	,,	35
Lentil	.. .. ..	,,	199	,,	47
Lobster Bisque	..	,,	180	,,	42
Minestrone	..	,,	129	,,	30
Oxtail	.. .. ..	,,	185	,,	43
Pea & Ham	.. ..	,,	226	,,	53
Pheasant Consomme	..	,,	49	,,	11
Poacher's Broth	..	,,	177	,,	42
Royal Game	.. ..	,,	138	,,	32

Soups

Food	Quantities	Calories	Quantities	Calories
Salmon Bisque ..	1 can	180	100 g	42
Scotch Broth	,,	180	,,	42
Scotch Vegetable	,,	112	,,	26
Vichyssoise	,,	191	,,	45
CAMPBELLS *(canned, undiluted)* ..				
'Bumper Harvest Soups'				
Lentil	1 oz	13	100 g	47
Pea	,,	16	,,	57
Tomato	,,	17	,,	59
Average, all other flavours	,,	12	,,	42
'Condensed Soups'				
Beef Broth	,,	19	,,	68
Celery, Cream of ..	,,	14	,,	50
Chicken, Cream of ..	,,	28	,,	98
Chicken Rice	,,	14	,,	50
Consomme	,,	2	,,	8
Golden Vegetable ..	,,	13	,,	47
Lentil	,,	25	,,	88
Mushroom, Cream of ..	,,	24	,,	85
Oxtail	,,	24	,,	86
Pea & Ham	,,	35	,,	123
Scotch Broth	,,	20	,,	71
Stockpot	,,	16	,,	57
Tomato	,,	18	,,	65
Tomato, Cream of ..	,,	35	,,	123
Tomato Rice	,,	27	,,	96
Turkey & Vegetable Broth	,,	21	,,	76
Vegetable	,,	19	,,	67
'Granny's Soups'				
Chicken	,,	17	,,	60

Food	Quantities	Calories	Quantities	Calories
Chicken & Veg. Broth w/Rice	1 oz	10	100 g	37
Golden Pea w/Ham	,,	17	,,	59
Lentil	,,	16	,,	55
Macaroni Beef	,,	29	,,	102
Potato & Leek	,,	12	,,	43
Scotch Broth	,,	14	,,	50
Vegetable	,,	11	,,	38
Vegetable Broth w/Beef	,,	10	,,	35
Main Course Soups'				
Beef & Vegetable	,,	16	,,	56
Chicken & Vegetable	,,	14	,,	51
Ham, Turkey & Vegetables	,,	17	,,	60
Pea & Ham	,,	24	,,	86
Steak, Kidney & Vegetables	,,	16	,,	56
Superior Soups'				
Asparagus	,,	17	,,	61
Chicken & Sweetcorn	,,	25	,,	88
Consomme Madeira	,,	8	,,	29
Crab Bisque	,,	21	,,	74
French Onion	,,	8	,,	29
Goulash	,,	24	,,	86
Smoked Salmon, Cream of	,,	30	,,	106
CROSSE AND BLACKWELL *(canned)*				
Country Vegetable with Beef	1 oz	12	100 g	41
Cream of Chicken	,,	18	,,	63
Cream of Mushroom	,,	15	,,	54
Creamed Tomato	,,	20	,,	71
Farmhouse Thick Vegetable	,,	15	,,	53

Soups

Food	Quantities	Calories	Quantities	Calories
Scottish Lentil with Vegetable	1 oz	13	100 g	45
Minestrone	,,	14	,,	48
Oxtail	,,	14	,,	49
Oxtail & Vegetable	,,	11	,,	38
Scotch Broth	,,	18	,,	62
Vegetable	,,	14	,,	48
'Speciality Soups'				
Consomme	,,	6	,,	22
French Onion	,,	5	,,	18
Lobster Bisque	,,	11	,,	38
Vichyssoise	,,	13	,,	47
'Chef Chunky Soups'				
Beef Flavour	,,	16	,,	57
Tomato and Vegetable	,,	15	,,	52
Vegetable	,,	15	,,	53
Chicken	,,	14	,,	50
(Packet, reconstituted)				
Spring Vegetable	,,	4	,,	16
Tomato	,,	10	,,	36
Average all other flavours	,,	28	,,	8
HEINZ				
'Ready to Serve Soups'				
Beef Broth	1 oz	12	100 g	42
Beef Soup	,,	18	,,	63
Celery, cream of	,,	14	,,	49
Chicken, cream of	,,	17	,,	60
Farmhouse Thick Vegetable	,,	13	,,	46
Lentil	,,	17	,,	60
Minestrone	,,	12	,,	42
Mulligatawny	,,	17	,,	60

Food	Quantities	Calories	Quantities	Calories
Mushroom, cream of ..	1 oz	17	100 g	60
Oxtail	,,	14	,,	49
Pea & Ham	,,	19	,,	67
Scotch Broth	,,	11	,,	40
Scottish Vegetable with Lentils ..	,,	17	,,	60
Spring Vegetable ..	,,	12	,,	42
Tomato, Cream of ..	,,	22	,,	79
Vegetable	,,	15	,,	53
'Big Soups'				
Beef & Vegetable ..	,,	15	,,	53
Beef Broth	,,	16	,,	55
Chicken & Vegetable ..	,,	14	,,	48
Golden Vegetable ..	,,	12	,,	44
Minestrone	,,	16	,,	57
Vegetable	,,	15	,,	54
Vegetable & Lentil ..	,,	14	,,	48
'Soupermugs' (reconstituted)				
Beef & Tomato ..	,,	11	,,	38
Chicken	,,	14	,,	48
Golden Chicken with Noodles ..	,,	9	,,	31
Oxtail	,,	10	,,	37
Spring Vegetable ..	,,	9	,,	31
Tomato	,,	11	,,	38
'Ready to Serve'				
Golden Chicken & Mushroom	,,	15	,,	52
Golden Chicken & Vegetable	,,	11	,,	40
Golden Vegetable ..	,,	11	,,	39
INTERNATIONAL Chicken Soup	1 oz	18	100 g	63

Soups

Food		Quantities	Calories	Quantities	Calories
Farmhouse Vegetable	..	1 oz	14	100 g	53
Mushroom	.. ..	,,	14	,,	54
Oxtail	.. .. ..	,,	13	,,	49
Tomato	.. ..	,,	20	,,	71
Vegetable	.. ..	,,	13	,,	48
KNORR *(packet)*					
Asparagus	.. ..	1 packet	248	100 g	357
Chicken Noodle	..	,,	187	,,	347
Cornish Seafood	..	,,	278	,,	373
Country Mushroom	..	,,	331	,,	389
Crofters' Thick Vegetable		,,	250	,,	321
Farmhouse Chicken & Leek	..	,,	233	,,	337
Florida Spring Vegetable		,,	107	,,	281
French Onion	.. ..	,,	176	,,	325
Highland Lentil	..	,,	301	,,	314
Leek	.. .. ..	,,	307	,,	372
Minestrone	.. ..	,,	248	,,	314
Northumbrian Potato & Leek	..	,,	269	,,	330
Original Tomato	..	,,	312	,,	350
Oxtail	.. ..	,,	252	,,	329
Pea with Ham	.. ..	,,	206	,,	327
Thick Chicken Broth	..	,,	271	,,	348
Tomato & Beef	.. ..	,,	277	,,	340
Virginia Sweetcorn	..	,,	327	,,	367
'Hearty Soups'					
Boston Bean	.. ..	,,	270	,,	294
Farmhouse Vegetable & Beef	..	,,	228	,,	316
Highland Scotch Broth	..	,,	257	,,	323

Food	Quantities	Calories	Quantities	Calories
Maryland with Sweetcorn	1 packet	267	100 g	340
'Quick Soups'				
Asparagus	1 cup	84	—	—
Chicken	"	90	—	—
Chicken & Leek	"	88	—	—
Chicken & Mushroom	"	80	—	—
French Onion	"	63	—	—
Golden Vegetable	"	84	—	—
Oxtail	"	65	—	—
Pea with Ham	"	70	—	—
Sweetcorn	"	83	—	—
Tomato	"	99	—	—
'Special Recipe Quick Soups'				
Chicken & Ham w/Croutons	"	97	—	—
Country Vegetable w/Croutons	"	87	—	—
French Onion w/Croutons	"	83	—	—
Minestrone w/croutons	1 cup	80	—	—
MARKS AND SPENCER *(canned)*				
Cream of Chicken	1 oz	17	100 g	60
Cream of Mushroom	"	14	"	50
Cream of Tomato	"	16	"	55
Golden Vegetable	"	10	"	37
Oxtail	"	12	"	44
OXO *(cubes)*				
Chicken Oxo	1 oz	60	100 g	210
Oxo Beef Drink	"	28	"	100
Red Oxo	"	70	"	245

Soups

Food		Quantities	Calories	Quantities	Calories
SAFEWAY *(canned)*					
Cream of Chicken	..	1 oz	15	100 g	52
Cream of Mushroom/					
Tomato	..	,,	19	,,	68
Oxtail ..	.. ..	,,	12	,,	43
Scotch Broth	.. ..	,,	12	,,	43
Vegetable	.. ..	,,	11	,,	39
(packet as sold)					
Asparagus	.. ..	,,	106	,,	373
Chicken Noodle	..	,,	91	,,	320
Golden Vegetable	..	,,	96	,,	338
Minestrone	.. ..	,,	92	,,	323
Mushroom	.. ..	,,	101	,,	355
Oxtail ..	.. ..	,,	99	,,	350
Spring Vegetable	..	,,	90	,,	317
Thick Chicken	..	,,	99	,,	350
Tomato	.. ..	,,	96	,,	339
(Soup-In-A-Cup as sold)					
Beef & Tomato	..	,,	100	,,	354
Chicken	.. ..	,,	112	,,	395
Golden Vegetable	..	,,	103	,,	363
Tomato	.. ..	,,	96	,,	338
TESCO *(canned)*					
Cream of Chicken	..	1 oz	15	100 g	54
Cream of Mushroom	..	,,	16	,,	55
Cream of Tomato	..	,,	10	,,	36
Oxtail ..	.. ..	,,	15	,,	54
Vegetable	.. ..	,,	10	,,	35
(packet as sold)					
Asparagus	.. ..	,,	104	,,	365
Chicken Noodle	.. ..	,,	105	,,	368

Food		Quantities	Calories	Quantities	Calories
French Style Onion	..	1 oz	66	100 g	234
Minestrone	.. ..	,,	103	,,	362
Mushroom	.. ..	,,	103	,,	362
Oxtail	.. .. ..	,,	94	,,	330
Pea & Ham	.. ..	,,	110	,,	386
Scotch Broth	.. ..	,,	98	,,	345
Spring Vegetable	..	,,	66	,,	234
Tomato	.. ..	,,	99	,,	348
WAITROSE					
Chicken, cream of	..	1 oz	15	100 g	53
Lobster	.. ..	,,	19	,,	67
Mushroom, Cream of	..	,,	14	,,	49
Oxtail	.. .. ..	,,	9	,,	32
Scotch Broth	.. ..	,,	11	,,	39
Tomato, Cream of	..	,,	15	,,	53
Vegetable	.. ..	,,	14	,,	49

Sweets & Chocolates

Some people will argue that this section should not be in this book at all! They will say that anybody who has any kind of weight problem should not even think of these foods ever again. I do not agree. Most of us, at some time or another, crave a bar of chocolate. Once your ideal weight has been achieved there is no reason why you should not have one as long as it is counted in your daily calorie allowance. Where manufacturers have supplied the calories per bar these have been included. However, as the weight of the bars does change from year to year the calories per 100 g has also been included.

Food	Quantities	Calories	Quantities	Calories
CADBURY'S				
(Chocolate Products)				
Bar 6	1 bar	220	100 g	545
Bournville				
50 g	,	260	,,	515
100 g	,,	515	—	—
Brazilnut, 100 g	,,	550	—	—
Caramel	,,	245	100 g	490
Creme Eggs	1 egg	170	,,	435
Crunchie,				
Small	1 bar	95	,,	470

Food	Quantities	Calories	Quantities	Calories
Large	1 bar	165	—	—
Curly Wurly	,,	130	100 g	450
Dairy Milk,				
60 g	1 bar	315	,,	525
125 g	,,	660	—	—
Dipped Flake	,,	145	,,	535
Double Decker	,,	230	,,	450
Flake	,,	180	,,	525
Fruit & Nut,				
Standard	,,	270	,,	470
100 g	,,	470	—	—
Fudge	,,	135	100 g	440
Hazel Whirls	1 carton	1755	,,	540
Milk Chocolate Buttons				
Large	1 packet	250	,,	525
Standard	,,	160	—	—
Mini Eggs	—		100 g	500
Mixed Nuts	—	—	,,	545
Picnic	1 bar	230	,,	500
Roast Almond	—	—	,,	540
Star Bar	1 bar	270	,,	505
Chocolate Assortments)				
Bournville Selection	—	—	,,	465
Contrast	—	—	,,	450
Milk Tray	—	—	,,	455
Roses	—	—	,,	445
RY				
Chocolate Cream	1 bar	210	100 g	415
Turkish Delight	,,	190	,,	360

Sweets and Chocolates

Food	Quantities	Calories	Quantities	Calorie
(Chocolate Products)				
Cream Filled Bars, all flavours ..	1 oz	119	100 g	420
Hazelnut Toffee Nougat ..	,,	139	,,	490
Honeycomb Crunch ..	,,	174	,,	614
Liquer Bars, all flavours ..	,,	132	,,	467
Milk Wafer Bar ..	,,	145	,,	510
Mini Sticks,				
Mint	,,	135	,,	477
Mocca	,,	157	,,	552
Hazelnut	,,	156	,,	550
Swiss,				
Milk	,,	151	,,	533
Plain	,,	149	,,	524
Soft Filled Milk ..	,,	174	,,	614
(Non-Chocolate Products)				
Assorted Fruit Drops ..	,,	102	,,	360
Assorted Fruit Sweets ..	,,	107	,,	378
Butter Toffee Bon-Bons ..	,,	108	,,	380
Chews, bag	,,	109	,,	381
Chews, Stick pack ..	,,	104	,,	368
Catherine Wheels ..	,,	88	,,	310
Dolly Mixtures ..	,,	110	,,	387
Double Devon Toffees ..	,,	125	,,	440
Fruit Flavoured Assortment ..	,,	99	,,	350
Jaffa Assortment ..	,,	99	,,	350
Liquorice Sticks ..	,,	110	,,	389
Liquorice Allsorts ..	,,	104	,,	368
Lollipops	,,	109	,,	385
Mini Wine Gums ..	,,	97	,,	342
Mint Imperials ..	,,	105	,,	370
Mintoes	,,	116	,,	410

Food	Quantities	Calories	Quantities	Calories
Nutty Toffee Puffs	1 oz	125	100 g	439
Popcorn	,,	95	,,	334
Praline Eclairs	,,	133	,,	470
Soft Mints	,,	104	,,	365
Wine Gums	,,	97	,,	342
MARS				
(Chocolate Products)				
Banjo	1 bar	123	—	—
Bounty, milk & plain	single	150	—	—
Galaxy	1 oz	152	100 g	535
Galaxy counters	each	6	—	—
Maltesers	small bag	179	,,	497
Maltesers	small box	740	,,	497
Marathon	1 bar	308	—	—
Marathon fun size	,,	97	—	—
Mars bar	each	326	—	—
Mars bar, fun size	each	90	—	—
Milky Way	,,	139	—	—
Milky Way, fun size	each	76	—	—
Revels	small bag	182	100 g	496
Ripple	each	141	—	—
Topic	,,	287	—	—
Treets, peanut	small bag	248	100 g	516
Treets, toffee	,,	250	,,	516
Twix	single	137	—	—
(Non Chocolate Products)				
Glees	1 pack	206	100 g	514
Lockets	,,	154	,,	355
Minstrels	small bag	217	—	—
Opals & Pacers	each	21	—	—

Sweets and Chocolates

Food	Quantities	Calories	Quantities	Calories
Spangles	1 pack	144	—	—
Tunes, cherry & honey ..	,,	145	—	—
PASCALL				
Fruit Bonbons ..	1 packet	425	100 g	370
Fruit Pastilles	,,	410	,,	315
Marshmallows ..	,,	410	,,	320
Milk Chocolate Eclairs ..	,,	490	,,	440
Murraymints	,,	500	,,	410
ROWNTREE MACINTOSH *(Chocolate Products)*				
Aero, all flavours ..	1 oz	150	100 g	525
After Eight Mints	1 sweet	35	,,	420
Blue Riband	each	105	,,	540
Breakaway, Milk ..	,,	105	,,	525
Cabana	,,	255	,,	445
Caramac, medium ..	,,	155	,,	555
Caramel Wafer ..	,,	85	,,	460
Drifter	1 biscuit	115	,,	460
Golden Cup, small ..	small bar	105	,,	475
Kit Kat	1 finger	55	,,	505
Lion Bar	each	215	,,	490
Matchmakers	,,	7	,,	485
Matchmakers, long ..	,,	20	,,	485
Mintola	1 sweet	25	,,	440
Montego, ginger ..	each	120	,,	520
Munchies	1 sweet	25	,,	505
Nutty	each	255	,,	500
Prize	,,	225	,,	450
Rolo	1 sweet	25	,,	450
Smarties	small tube	155	,,	460

Food	Quantities	Calories	Quantities	Calories
Splicer	each	180	100 g	420
Texan	,,	180	,,	420
Toffee Crisp	,,	195	,,	510
Walnut whip, all flavours	,,	167	,,	475
Yorkie,				
Milk	1 oz	150	,,	525
Raisin & Biscuit	,,	133	,,	470
Peanut	,,	155	,,	545
Non Chocolate Products)				
Fox's Glacier Fruits,				
stickpack	1 sweet	12	,,	365
Fox's Glacier Fruits, bag	,,	20	,,	365
Fox's Glacier Mints,				
stickpack	,,	12	,,	380
Fox's Glacier Mints, bag	,,	20	,,	380
Fruit Gums	,,	2	,,	195
Fruit Pastilles	,,	10	,,	320
Polo Mints	,,	6	,,	400
Toffees, assorted	,,	30	,,	430
Toffee, golden	,,	30	,,	475
Toffo, all flavours	,,	20	,,	425
Tooty Frooties & Minties	,,	8	,,	410
Tots,				
Bunnytots	1 bag	190	,,	420
Candytots	,,	180	,,	400
Jellytots	,,	170	,,	350
TESCO				
Butterkist Popcorn	1 oz	111	100 g	390
Butterscotch, boiled	,,	89	,,	121
Chewy Fruit	,,	106	,,	375

Sweets and Chocolates

Food	Quantities	Calories	Quantities	Calories
Chocolate Coated,				
Brazils	1 oz	142	100 g	500
Eclairs	,,	124	,,	437
Peanuts	,,	153	,,	540
Peanuts & Raisins ..	,,	136	,,	480
Toffee Rolls ..	,,	128	,,	452
Fudge	,,	109	,,	385
Liquorice,				
Allsorts	,,	103	,,	363
Novelties	,,	97	,,	341
Marshmallows ..	,,	88	,,	310
Sparkling,				
Fruits & Mints ..	,,	105	,,	370
Toffee,				
Assortment	,,	136	,,	480
Brazils	,,	119	,,	420
Cream	,,	133	,,	470
WAITROSE				
Butterscotch	1 oz	113	100 g	398
Chocolate Assortment ..	,,	21	,,	468
Clear Fruits & Mints ..	,,	93	,,	327
Devon Toffees	,,	123	,,	433
Fruit Jellies	,,	73	,,	257
Liquorice Allsorts ..	,,	90	,,	317
Orange & Lemon Slices	,,	93	,,	327

Vegetables

Vegetables are very low in calories. In fact, the calorie content of many fresh vegetables is negligible and they can therefore be eaten in large quantities without any weight gain resulting. In this edition vegetables with less than 25 calories per 100 g have been omitted. Vegetables are also a source of many essential vitamins. Potatoes—although higher in calories—are of considerable nutritional value and the skins, as is now well known, are a good source of fibre. However, if you are trying to lose weight, beware of fried potatoes. Dried vegetables and pulses are also fibre-rich but they should be carefully weighed and the calories counted.

Food		Quantities	Calories	Quantities	Calories
BATCHELOR					
(canned)					
Cannellini Beans	..	223 g	152	100 g	68
Butter Beans	.. ..	223 g	151	„	68
Mushy Peas	.. ..	304 g	246	„	81
Processed Peas	..	304 g	194	„	64
(cooking aids)					
Mixed Peppers	..	46 g	136	—	—
Mixed Vegetable Jar	..	53 g	145	—	—
Sliced Onion Jar	..	53 g	167	—	—

Vegetables

Food	Quantities	Calories	Quantities	Calories
Quick Soak Peas	254 g	719	100 g	285
Surprise Peas	62 g	178	,,	110
Surprise Beans ..	33 g	89	—	—
BAXTER *(canned)*				
Beets, Diced & Shredded ..	—	—	100 g	45
Beets, Sliced	—	—	,,	30
BIRD'S EYE *(frozen)*				
Corn on the Cob ..	7 oz	140	—	—
'Potato Products'				
Bubble 'n Squeak ..	1 patty	50	—	—
Chips	1 oz	40	100 g	141
Crispy Potato Fritters ..	,,	40	,,	141
Croquette Potatoes ..	one	40	—	—
Oven Chips	1 oz	45	100 g	158
Oven Stars	,,	65	,,	229
Potato Waffles ..	one	80	—	—
Mini Waffles	,,	23	—	—
Rice, Peas and Mushrooms ..	1 oz	40	100 g	141
Rice, Sweetcorn & Peppers ..	,,	40	,,	141
Small Onions and White Sauce ..	5 oz packet	200	—	—
Sweet Corn	1 oz	30	100 g	106
BUITONI *(canned)*				
Ratatouille	1 can	146	—	—
CADBURY *(instant)*				
Smash,				
as sold	1 oz	94	100 g	330
reconstituted ..	,,	18	,,	65

Food	Quantities	Calories	Quantities	Calories
CROSSE AND BLACKWELL				
'Pot Soups'				
Country Chicken & Leek	1 sachet	62	—	—
Farmhouse Potato & Veg.	,,	65	—	—
Harvest Vegetable & Beef	,,	74	—	—
Rich Tomato	,,	78	—	—
FINDUS (*frozen*)				
Broad Beans	1 oz	15	100 g	53
Broccoli Spears ..	,,	9	,,	32
Chips	,,	31	,,	109
Corn on the Cob ..	,,	36	,,	127
Country Mix	,,	16	,,	55
Garden Mix	,,	13	,,	46
Green Beans	,,	8	,,	30
Grill Chips	,,	40	,,	144
Haricot Verts	,,	19	,,	67
Mixed Vegetables ..	,,	17	,,	59
Parsnips	,,	14	,,	49
Peas	,,	15	,,	53
Petits Pois	,,	18	,,	63
Potato Croquettes ..	,,	26	,,	91
Potatoes, Sautés ..	,,	28	,,	97
Spinach, chopped ..	,,	9	,,	31
Spinach, whole leaf ..	,,	9	,,	31
Summer Harvest Mix ..	,,	20	,,	72
Sweetcorn	,,	36	,,	127
Swiss Style Potatoes ..	,,	23	,,	80
GREEN GIANT (*canned*)				
Cream Style Corn ..	10 oz can	255	100 g	85
Mexicorn	7 oz can	170	,,	86

Vegetables

Food	Quantities	Calories	Quantities	Calories
Niblets	7 oz can	165	100 g	83
(frozen)				
Corn on the Cob & Nibble	—	—	,,	88
Niblets Corn	—	—	,,	83
INTERNATIONAL *(canned)*				
Garden Peas	—	—	100 g	46
Marrowfat Processed Peas	—	—	,,	80
New Potatoes	—	—	,,	64
Processed Peas	—	—	,,	73
(frozen)				
Oven Chips	—	—	,,	158
Peas & Minted Peas	—	—	,,	53
MARKS AND SPENCER *(frozen)*				
Broccoli, Stir Fry	—	—	100 g	29
Cauliflower Cheese	—	—	,,	149
Cauliflower, Stir Fry	—	—	,,	45
Chips, Crinkle Cut	—	—	,,	109
Chips, Just Bake	—	—	,,	208
Leeks with Cheese Sauce	—	—	,,	127
Petits Pois	—	—	,,	53
Petits Pois a la Francaise	—	—	,,	65
Sliced Potato Bake	—	—	,,	107
Whole Beans	—	—	,,	35
PRINCES				
Sweetcorn, drained	1 oz	21	,,	76
ROSS *(frozen)*				
Broad Beans	1 oz	20	100 g	70
Broccoli Spears	,,	7	,,	25

Food	Quantities	Calories	Quantities	Calories
Brussels Sprouts	1 oz	11	100 g	39
Cabbage, shredded ..	,,	8	,,	30
Carrots	,,	7	,,	25
Casserole Mix	,,	7	,,	25
Cauliflower Florets ..	,,	7	,,	25
Country Mix	,,	7	,,	25
Farmhouse Mix ..	,,	11	,,	40
Green Beans	,,	10	,,	35
Mixed Vegetables ..	,,	16	,,	56
Onion Ringers ..	,,	65	,,	230
Peas	,,	23	,,	81
Potato Products				
Bubble & Squeak ..	,,	17	,,	60
Crinkle Cut Chips ..	,,	40	,,	140
Croquettes	,,	31	,,	110
Hash Browns ..	,,	23	,,	80
Jacket Chips ..	,,	34	,,	120
Jacket Scallops ..	,,	34	,,	120
Noisettes	,,	54	,,	190
Oven Chips	,,	43	,,	150
Oven Crunches ..	,,	43	,,	150
Steak Chips	,,	31	,,	110
Straight Cut Chips ..	,,	34	,,	120
Waffles	,,	57	,,	200
Special Mix	,,	16	,,	55
Spinach	,,	9	,,	30
Spring Greens	,,	7	,,	25
Stewpack	,,	7	,,	25
Stir Fry	,,	17	,,	60
Swede	,,	6	,,	21
Sweetcorn	,,	31	,,	110
Turnip	,,	6	,,	21

Vegetables

Food	Quantities	Calories	Quantities	Calories
SAFEWAY *(canned)*				
Broad Beans	—	—	100 g	34
Butter Beans	—	—	,,	59
Garden Peas	—	—	,,	60
Marrowfat Peas ..	—	—	,,	78
Processed Peas ..	—	—	,,	80
(frozen)				
Chips, Potato	—	—	,,	140
Chips, Oven	—	—	,,	150
SPAR				
Easy Chips *(frozen)* ..	—	—	100 g	208
Instant Potato	—	—	1 serving	90
TESCO *(canned)*				
Broad Beans	—	—	100 g	49
Butter Beans	—	—	,,	95
Garden Peas	—	—	,,	60
Jersey Potatoes ..	—	—	,,	78
Kidney Beans	—	—	,,	121
Marrowfat Peas ..	—	—	,,	78
Mixed Vegetables ..	—	—	,,	46
Mushy Peas	—	—	,,	243
Pease Pudding ..	—	—	,,	90
Petits Pois	—	—	,,	52
Processed Peas ..	—	—	,,	78
Summer Mixed Vegetables ..	—	—	,,	321
Sweetcorn/Sweetcorn & Peppers ..	—	—	,,	108
Ratatouille	—	—	,,	33

Food		Quantities	Calories	Quantities	Calories
(dried)					
Instant Mashed Potato	..	1 oz	93	100 g	327
Mixed Peppers	..	,,	58	,,	205
Mixed Vegetables	..	,,	92	,,	325
Peas,					
Garden	.. ..	,,	77	,,	270
Marrowfat	.. ..	,,	118	,,	414
Yellow Split	..	,,	89	,,	314
Mushrooms	.. ..	,,	92	,,	325
Onions, Sliced	..	,,	84	,,	296
Tomato Whirls	..	,,	91	,,	320
(Frozen)					
Chips,					
Crinkle	.. ..	,,	56	,,	198
Oven	.. ..	,,	43	,,	150
Straight Cut	..	,,	56	,,	198
Special Mixed Vegetables		—	—	,,	68
Sprouts	.. ..	—	—	,,	35
WAITROSE					
(canned)					
Beetroot & Baby Beetroot		1 oz	13	100 g	46
Broad Beans	.. ..	,,	12	,,	42
Butter Beans	.. ..	,,	28	,,	98
Garden Peas	.. ..	,,	14	,,	49
Marrowfat Peas	..	,,	27	,,	95
Potatoes & Jersey Potatoes		,,	21	,,	74
(dried)					
Butter Beans	.. ..	,,	76	,,	267
Lentils	.. ..	,,	84	,,	295
Peas	.. .. ..	,,	78	,,	278
Quick Dried & Split Peas	..	,,	86	,,	303

Vegetables

Food	Quantities	Calories	Quantities	Calories
(frozen)				
Broccoli	1 oz	9	100 g	32
Brussels Sprouts	,,	9	,,	32
Peas	,,	18	,,	63
Potato Products				
American Fries, fried ..	,,	79	,,	278
Chips, crinkle cut, fried ..	,,	61	,,	215
Oven Chips, baked or grilled ..	,,	61	,,	215
Oven Chips, grilled ..	,,	50	,,	176
Straight cut chips, fried ..	,,	63	,,	222

See over for further slimming
publications by Marina Andrews and
Katy Parks.

ENCYCLOPAEDIA OF SLIMMING DIETS

— Marina Andrews —

"You're bound to find just the right diet for you." VOGUE

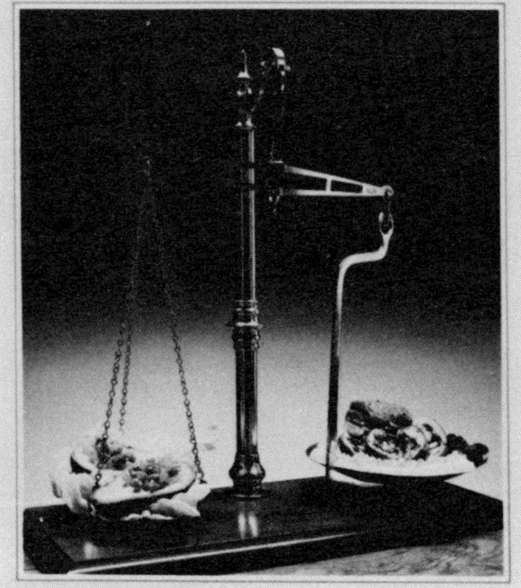

Paperback £4.95
ISBN 0 85140 608 4

The Encyclopaedia of Slimming Diets tells you all you need to know about safe and healthy slimming. 176 diets are arranged in categories according to their length — from twenty-four hours for those with just a few pounds to lose to two months for more drastic weight loss.

An enormous variety of diets caters for all tastes, from apple and cheese to lettuce and peach or a South American health drink. All have been extensively tested by the author and her clients.

All the diets are devised by slimming expert, Marina Andrews, who runs London's famous Town and Country Health Club. She regularly writes for *Vogue* and the *Sunday Express*.

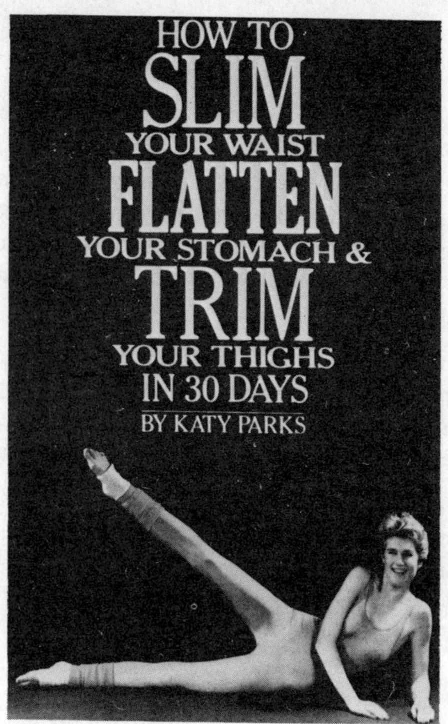

Paperback £1.95
ISBN 0 85140 612 2

How To Slim Your Waist, Flatten Your Stomach & Trim Your Thighs In 30 Days — The simple plan for a slimmer, trimmer, more beautiful body in just 30 days!

Katy Parks, a Southern Californian teaching at London's Pineapple Dance Studios invites you to get your whole body in shape with her specially-devised three part programme. The 30-day regime sets out an easy-to-follow exercise routine with essential advice on aerobic exercise and diet. It is fully illustrated with photographs of Katy performing all the exercises.

The Arlington Pocket Books

The ABC Of Vitamins
Pocket Guide To Allergies
The Anti-Acne Book
Pocket Guide To Back Pain
Pocket Calorie Guide To Branded Foods
Pocket Calorie Guide To Safe Slimming
The Carbohydrate Counter
The Carbohydrate Counter For Branded Foods
The Cholesterol Counter
Pocket Guide To Cystitis
Pocket A To Z Guide To Freezing Food
The Pocket Gourmet Book I: Soups
Herbs And Spices
The Menopause Questions And Answers
Pocket Guide To Migraines And Headaches
The Sodium Counter
Pocket A To Z Guide To Stain Removal
Pocket Guide To Stress
The Ten Best Diets In The World
A Parent's Guide To Toilet Training
Where Do I Come From?
Pocket Guide To Yoga For Weight Control